150 Pounds Gone

FOREVER

150 Pounds Gone
FOREVER

How I Lost Half My Size and You Can Too

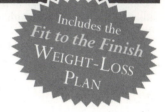

Includes the
Fit to the Finish
WEIGHT-LOSS
PLAN

DIANE CARBONELL

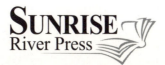

SUNRISE
River Press

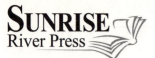

Sunrise River Press
39966 Grand Avenue
North Branch, MN 55056
Phone: 651-277-1400 or 800-895-4585
Fax: 651-277-1203
www.sunriseriverpress.com

Edit by Karen Chernyaev
Layout by Monica Seiberlich

ISBN 978-1-934716-41-0
Item No. SRP641

Library of Congress Cataloging-in-Publication Data

Carbonell, Diane,
  150 pounds gone forever / by Diane Carbonell.
    p. cm.
  ISBN 978-1-934716-41-0
  1. Carbonell, Diane, 1965–Health. 2. Overweight persons–Biography.
3. Weight loss. 4. Physical fitness for women. I. Title. II. Title:
One hundred fifty pounds gone forever.
  RC628.C373 2012
  613.7'12–dc23
                                    2011051763

Printed in USA
10 9 8 7 6 5 4 3 2 1

Dedication

To my wonderful husband, John, who supported me when
I needed it most, and to my seven lovely children

Contents

Acknowledgments

This book would not have been possible without the help of my family, my supportive agent Linda Konner, my understanding editor Karen Chernyaev, and all the friends who encouraged me to keep writing and never give up.

Foreword

More than two-thirds of Americans are overweight or obese and need to lose weight to optimize health. Dieting, however, has never been easy. If your experience is similar to many of my new clients, you have probably tried countless diets but never learned how to eat successfully. The goal of any successful weight-loss plan should be to lose weight safely and realistically while learning how to eat the foods you love in reasonable portions. Diane Carbonell's *150 Pounds Gone Forever* shows you how to do just that. It is practical, realistic, and safe and leaves lots of room for flexibility. Whether you would like to lose 10 pounds, 50 pounds, or more, this program delivers a painless way to put you on the road to health and *permanent* weight loss.

Diane Carbonell is an inspiration to anyone trying to lose weight and keep it off. She lost more than 150 pounds and has kept the weight off. You can too. Diane details her heartwarming personal challenges, which just about any overweight individual can relate to. She offers a positive approach toward eating and focuses on wellness and health in addition to weight loss. In this book, Diane doesn't just tell you what you can't eat; she tells you what you can eat. And best of all, this plan is based on successful results she has seen on herself.

150 Pounds Gone Forever offers a three-pronged approach to weight loss that is sensible and that works: limiting fat, controlling portion size, and engaging in a realistic exercise program. It is a real-life sensible plan. In my experience, as a nutritionist who has counseled overweight individuals for more than twenty-five years, this is an excellent approach to losing weight and keeping it off. This book contains no gimmicks, fad diets, or special products that promise "instant" results—as they do not exist. Many diets deprive your body of vital nutrients while omitting entire food groups. *150 Pounds Gone Forever* provides solid information on nutrition and guidelines endorsed by leading health authorities. It comes at a time when we are bombarded by so many diet plans, most of which work for only the short run.

What's the point in losing weight if you are not going to keep it off? Clearly, there is none. *150 Pounds Gone Forever* will start you on the road to successful weight loss as well as weight maintenance. It encourages you to eat from all the food groups, to include portion-controlled amounts of your favorite foods, and to engage in a regular exercise program that works for you. In my opinion, this is the only way to lose weight and keep it off. Diane Carbonell will teach you how to make simple, painless changes in your diet and lifestyle that will help you shed pounds permanently. Read on and learn how to lose weight realistically and keep it off forever.

Enjoy!

Lisa R. Young, PhD, RD, CDN, is the author of *The Portion Teller Plan: The No-Diet Reality Guide to Eating, Cheating, and Losing Weight Permanently.*

Introduction

Ever since I lost 158 pounds, I've had the desire to help people who feel stuck in a body they no longer recognize. I currently write a blog, which you can find at www.fittothefinish.com/blog, and I teach weight-loss classes based on my weight-loss plan, Fit to the Finish. Over the years, I have witnessed other people have the same kind of success I've had. This book honors the many requests I've had to put my story and my plan together in a book anyone can use to get results.

If you have ever stood in front of your mirror wondering how you got to be overweight, this book is for you. Like you, I tried many different diet plans in an attempt to lose weight, but nothing clicked for me. As I stood in front of my mirror in 1997, I realized that the person looking back at me bore little resemblance to the person I wanted to be. At more than 300 pounds, I was depressed and unattractive. I suffered from low self-esteem and had little energy. I knew in my heart that the only way to overcome my all-consuming overeating was to make some changes.

I did not want a quick fix. I'd had my share of unsuccessful dieting experiences and was tired of bouncing from one fad diet to the next. I knew I didn't need a short-term weight-loss plan but one that would last a lifetime.

In *150 Pounds Gone Forever,* I detail my personal challenges of living as an obese wife, mother, and friend. I give you a picture of a life lived in morbid obesity (all while keeping a sense of humor) and the amazing, dramatic changes that came about as I lost weight and found myself again. It was not all roses and happiness, as I had to deal with difficult life situations, unexpected reactions from friends and family, and the fear that I might regain every single pound I lost.

This book is part memoir and part self-help, as I weave together stories of my life with questions just for you. You will have the opportunity to examine why you are overweight, to determine what kinds of foods push your buttons, and to develop lifelong weight-maintenance strategies that will work for you. I also give you a three-pronged approach to losing weight that is easy, costs very little, and works.

At first you will learn to eat according to established medical guidelines, practice eating the correct portions of food, and begin a realistic exercise program. As you journey with me through *150 Pounds Gone Forever,* I will teach you how to deal with the daily weight-loss challenges that occur in each of our lives—from eating small portions during holidays to ordering a plan-friendly meal at a restaurant.

Is it easy? No, losing weight and keeping it off is not easy, but it is possible and sometimes even enjoyable. When I was stuffing my face with potato chips, or sitting down gingerly in chairs that might not hold my weight, I never in a million years imagined that I could lose half my weight and live the rest of my life as an active mom to seven beautiful children. Instead, I imagined myself sitting in a chair while the rest of my family enjoyed hikes, bike rides, running in the yard, and swimming. Instead of envisioning myself running down the road with the wind in my hair, I imagined myself getting my shopping done on a grocery store scooter, oblivious to onlookers as I drove through the aisles picking out cookies, candy, and chips.

My first step out from the oppression of obesity involved realizing that I would never get closer to any dream by just sitting down and waiting for something to happen magically. Your first step may be reading this book, but your journey to lose weight and stay at a healthy weight for the rest of your life will involve many steps. You can start by answering the questions I pose in the upcoming chapters, making a commitment to healthy eating, learning to eat the right portion sizes, and starting an exercise program that fits within your lifestyle and physical capabilities.

The plan I offer isn't full of silver bullets and false hope. It's a practical and realistic plan grounded in common sense and sound medical information. I know that it can be scary to try to lose weight, as you might have failed before. But I assure you that you will never regret making the smart choice between a healthy and an unhealthy lifestyle. Never once when I was losing weight did I regret turning down a brownie or having a salad instead of a fatty hamburger. And never once was I sorry that I exercised.

As you begin your journey for the first or fiftieth time, remember that this can be your final weight-loss attempt. Once you successfully lose weight using Fit to the Finish and keep it off, you never have to go down the weight-loss road again. Instead, you can go through the rest of your life focusing on keeping your family relationships healthy, achieving your professional goals, and enjoying the satisfaction of knowing that you've already done the hard work you needed to do to keep your weight at a healthy level.

Whether you read this book in one sitting or take several months to work through the plan, refer back to the individual chapters often when you are faced with tempting foods, difficult social situations, or the inevitable birthday cakes and holiday cookies. I will show you that losing weight is not a short-term journey but a long-term, rewarding, and attainable lifestyle.

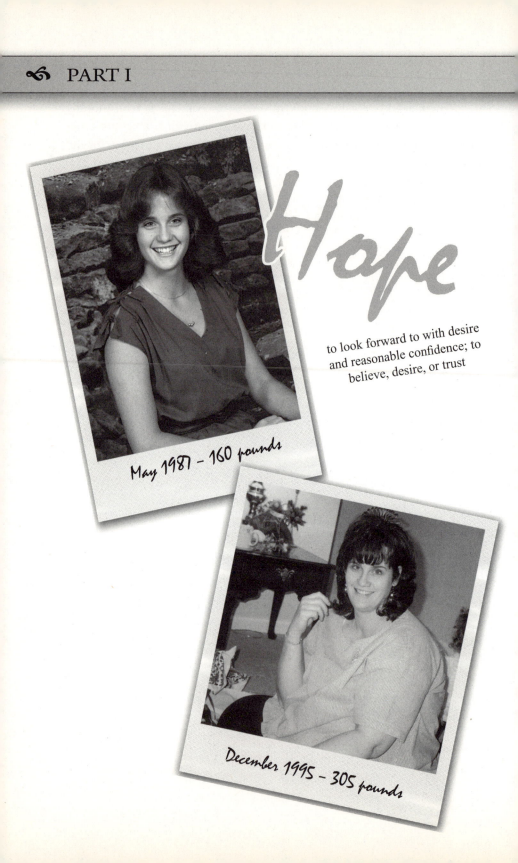

PART I

Hope

to look forward to with desire
and reasonable confidence; to
believe, desire, or trust

May 1987 – 160 pounds

December 1995 – 305 pounds

My Story

Welcome to my life as an overweight woman. Not all overweight people feel jolly and happy all the time, and I was one of them. I may have occasionally portrayed the jolly spirit in front of other people, but inside I usually felt angst over my appearance and my weight.

If you are overweight, you may see yourself in some of these stories. I empathize with the pain of being overweight and share my stories to let you know that I have been where you are.

My weight was but one facet of who I was, but that one facet had the power to overshadow other parts of my life. I allowed my weight to define how I felt about myself in social situations, how I felt about my relationship with my husband, and how I pictured my future.

My desire is that my story will give you a sense of hope and purpose. I will prove that you can lose a substantial amount of weight without appearing in front of millions of people on a television weight-loss show, having drastic weight-loss surgery, or spending a lot of money on special programs. If I can lose the 150 pounds that held me down, you can too.

Hello, Fatty

CLUNK. It seemed to be the loudest sound I had ever heard. I watched in horror as the nurse's thin fingers lifted the scale's 50-pound metal weight and moved it from 200 to 250 pounds. She then quickly adjusted the smaller measurement until the scale showed a number right below 300 pounds. Standing there, trying desperately not to look at the nurse, I was facing reality for the first time in years.

Earlier, in the waiting room, trying not to notice my thighs sticking out from under the arms of the chair, I had vainly tried to think of a way to avoid standing on that loathsome scale. Aside from running back to my car, nothing came to mind, so I reluctantly followed the nurse down the long hall, trying to decide whether it would be more embarrassing to take my shoes off or to weigh one pound more by leaving them on.

I leaned over, feeling my huge stomach squash against my thighs, and took off my shoes. As I removed them, I told the nurse with utmost sincerity, "These shoes are really heavy."

She nodded knowingly and proceeded to set the scale. After scratching the weight down on my chart, she cheerfully said, "Come with me." I waddled after her, trying to keep up with her quick pace. She left me alone in the exam room, where all I could do was anticipate the horrible, terrible things my doctor might say about my weight.

With the clunk of the scale still echoing in my head, I felt frightened, alone, and fat. Sitting on the exam table, my heart felt nearly as heavy as my body had on the scale. How had I come to be this overweight, underactive, lazy, morbidly obese woman? I had reached the upper limits of plus-size clothing and had resorted to making my own tent-shaped jumper dresses. My eating was out of control. I had a failed career as a dieter. The ever-widening girth of my hips had gotten me stuck in furniture, and I now required a seat belt extender. My three young children, ages seven, four, and three months, were on the move, and I was lagging far behind, needing to sit down and catch my breath after the slightest bit of activity. As much as the clunking weight scared me, the thought of missing out on the rest of my life frightened me more.

As I waited for the doctor, I began to reflect on my situation and to contemplate what led me to this desperate point.

In the Beginning . . . Food

I wasn't always big, huge, and round. I was a normal-size toddler, child, and teenager. I could run around, swim, and enjoy an active life. How did I get to the point where walking to the mailbox was too much for me?

I wish I could blame it on my childhood. That seems a convenient thing to do these days. After all, I was adopted into a strict military family that expected perfection and quickly handled any deviations from the standard. However, as controlling as my parents were, the bad food choices I made were mine alone. My mother prepared healthy foods, served lots of vegetables, and insisted I stay active. By forcing me to get off the couch and go outside to play, she helped me stay at a normal weight. But when I got my driver's license and was able to escape the confines of the house, I discovered the joys of drive-through restaurants, candy aisles in the grocery store, and convenience foods. Before long, I found myself using all my babysitting money to buy candy, chips, and Coke.

I still remember standing in the candy aisle trying to decide which colorful package I would choose. Should I get the Starburst, the M&M's, or the Hershey's Miniatures? If I had enough money, I usually just bought them all. My mother would have had a fit if she knew I was eating all that junk, so I hid the packages in the back of my closet. I visited my stash whenever I felt stressed, lonely, or bored.

Hiding my growing backside was an ever-increasing challenge. My mother made remarks such as, "Boy, Diane, your butt is getting big." My father said, "I don't ever remember you being so huge." They even laughed when my little brother chimed in, "Diane, you are fat!" Their comments left me feeling like a failure, and I resolved to get back at them. I knew better than to argue, so I got even with them by eating more.

Freedom and Food

Although I really wanted to leave it behind, my ever-expanding backside followed me to college. I carried it with me as I explored the expansive selection of food in my new town: the Big Man Breakfast at Denny's and the pizza delivered right to my dorm room. It was wonderful to be free. Every Friday, just to celebrate the beginning of the weekend, my roommates and I would share a 1-pound bag of M&M's. I always kept a close eye on those friends, though, to make sure they were not eating too many. After all, they were my M&M's.

Though still adding weight on a regular basis, I did manage to meet the love of my life—not over a buffet line as you might imagine but in the shoe department of Sears. John and I spent our dating years eating fattening dinners and extra-large tubs of buttered movie popcorn.

John loved to eat, and I loved to bake. Just for fun, and because I wanted them, I often whipped up a batch of chocolate chip cookies (six dozen) and took half of them down to his apartment. I'd keep the other thirty-six cookies for myself, because I never knew when the urge for chocolate would strike. I always felt a little guilty accepting his compliments on my generosity, knowing I had the same number of cookies for myself right down the road. The guilt did not stop me from eating the cookies when I got back home though.

For me, food was recreation.

John and I got married in 1987, and at 5 foot 10, I weighed a respectable 165 pounds. I should have appreciated that weight a little more, because an enormous problem was looming right around the corner. But instead of enjoying my closet full of size 10s and size 12s, I wished I weighed less. But wishing while eating Breyer's mint chocolate chip ice cream sprinkled with crushed-up Oreo cookies didn't do a thing to make my dreams come true.

Although I would have strongly denied any emotional attachment to food, it had a stranglehold on me. As a newlywed, I still hid food in my closet. I had a secret stash of treats in my office drawer, and I found it almost impossible to avoid fast-food drive-through windows. I struggled to make real meals and realized that although I loved to bake, I hated to cook. Who wants to prepare chicken when you can make cake?

My lack of enthusiasm for cooking sent John and me out to eat almost every night. When we walked in the door of Bennigan's, our favorite restaurant, the servers practically fell over themselves helping us to our table. We were great eaters and generous tippers. We ate so much that I'm surprised we didn't get sick before leaving the restaurant.

More Food for Me

The restaurant meals, secret food drawer, and extra pantry in my closet caught up with me in a big way. Every time I went to the doctor for a checkup, I was surprised when I got on the scale. How in the world could I weigh 180 when last time I weighed 175? How dare he imply I should watch my weight? I watched it! I watched it go up and up. The pounds just seemed to come on by themselves. I could not admit that my destructive eating habits were causing the problem. I was in denial.

If I could not admit to myself that I had a weight problem, I certainly never admitted it to John. One time, though, I almost had to tell him what size I really wore.

I had become a master at hiding the size of my clothes. When John and I went shopping together, I would take three different sizes into the dressing room. When I came out, I'd announce, "I'm going to get this one!" I would pay, and he would be none the wiser that instead of a size 12, I had purchased the tight size 14.

During the second year of our marriage, we planned a mountain vacation to Georgia with two other couples. We were all excited about hiking, shopping, and white-water rafting. As I packed for the vacation, I realized with great chagrin that I did not have a pair of blue jeans that fit. I had pretty much stopped wearing jeans because mine had gotten too small. I needed jeans for the vacation, so I invented an excuse to buy a new pair.

I went into the living room and held up my old pair. I said, "These pants are out of style, and I'd really like another pair." Being the good husband that he was, John didn't blink an eye but said, "Sure, I'll go with you."

I shook my head, "I'll just run out real quick." So shopping I went. I started with a size 14 but quickly realized it wasn't going to work. I couldn't even get the pants over my hips. Surely, I thought, that brand ran small, so I tried another pair. No go. They were even worse. Eventually I found a pair of tight 16s and reluctantly bought them, swearing to myself that I was going to lose this marriage weight. Even as I paid the cashier, I could hear the echo of my mother's voice in my mind: *Diane, your butt is getting so big.*

Back at our duplex, I took a pair of scissors from my sewing kit and surreptitiously cut the size tags out of the jeans, so John would not know what size I had bought. Those pants were tight, but I suffered through the vacation with them. Here is a picture of me from that trip, with my fabulous, brand-new, size-16 jeans.

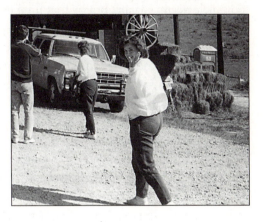

Once we returned from the trip, I joined Weight Watchers in a vain attempt to rid myself of the extra fat around my hips and thighs. Although I did lose some weight, I promptly gained it back the minute I stopped going to meetings. Weight Watchers works for some people, but I did not address any of my bad eating habits during my membership, so the weight loss was temporary and unsustainable.

Pregnancy and Food

I kept gaining and gaining, unable to control my eating habits. I was twenty-four when I got pregnant with my daughter Rachel and went from 196 to 271 pounds. Yes, you read right. I gained a whopping 75 pounds. Even my doctor couldn't believe it.

He was extremely concerned with my weight gain, particularly during my fifth month. I remember that appointment as if it were yesterday. The nurse weighed me and said I had gained 16 pounds since my last appointment. *Oh dear*, I thought.

I vividly recall my panic as the doctor came into the exam room with my chart in his hands. Would he notice? Would he say anything? He laid the chart on the counter, opened it up, and started reading. He stopped reading, turned away from the counter, took a step closer to me, and said in a shocked voice, "Did you really gain that much weight this month?" By the look on his face, I wasn't sure if he was shocked or impressed.

I shrugged and mumbled, "I guess so." I felt terrible inside. I knew it was too much weight to gain, but by that time I was completely out of control.

To his credit, he sent me to a very nice nutritionist, who told me that I should not gain any more weight for the duration of the pregnancy. I listened politely, took the food diary she gave me, and returned to work. I thought about what she had said and decided she really didn't know what she was talking about.

When I went back to see her two weeks later, empty food diary in hand, I had gained another 5 pounds. She was very concerned and gave me a firm lecture on the dangers of gaining too much weight during pregnancy, which included the baby becoming too large, gestational diabetes, and the likely difficulty of losing weight after the pregnancy. I listened with half an ear, trying to decide if I would have time to swing through Chick-fil-A, my favorite fast-food restaurant, on my way back to work. She scheduled me for another appointment, but I never went back.

The day of Rachel's birth, I weighed 271 pounds. In the hospital, I had to wear two gowns, one for the front and one for the back. It was humiliating to have the nurses place the elastic straps around my gigantic abdomen. They had a hard time finding baby Rachel's heartbeat under all the fat. Over and over, they would lose her heartbeat, not because she was in trouble but because my fat belly made it difficult for the transducer to pick up her heart tones. After a long labor, she was born and weighed in at a healthy 8 pounds, 2 ounces. The birth was an amazing experience. For the first time in my life, I knew someone who was related to me by blood.

Motherhood and Food

After Rachel's birth, I expected the 75 pounds to magically fall off. Many of my friends had "blown up" during pregnancy, only to shrink right back down after giving birth. I just assumed I would have the same experience, but I was wrong. Day after day, I weighed myself on my fancy Health o meter scale. After the first 25 pounds came off with no effort on my part, the scale stopped moving. I was so frustrated. Why wasn't I losing weight?

Three months after Rachel's birth, I was still wearing quickly fading maternity clothes. Instead of trying to diet, I drowned my frustration in food. I would load Rachel up into the car and drive to McDonald's nearly every day. The satisfaction of chocolate shakes, cheeseburgers, and fries made me feel better. But not for long.

Who was that woman I saw in the mirror? Where was the cute newly-wed, proud in her size-12 dress? I didn't recognize myself anymore. I felt despair when I saw my big chin, huge arms, and hips that wouldn't fit into a single clothing item I possessed—except the maternity jumpers. How did this happen to me?

Unable to deny reality any longer, in desperation I finally agreed to buy some new clothes. The wardrobe problem had hit the critical point. So John and I went shopping for a few things to "tide me over" until the weight started falling off.

We got to the department store, and John picked out some pants, shirts, and jumpers. I went into the dressing room and put on the first pair of size-16 pants. No go. Hmmm. I tried on a size-16 jumper and it got stuck around my armpits. I wiggled around trying to get the thing off. A shirt was the next futile attempt—it would not fit over my shoulders.

I was stuck in the dressing room. I didn't know what to do. How could I go out and tell John that none of the ugly big-girl clothes fit me? I could hear our daughter starting to make little baby noises, and I knew I had to do something. So I put my maternity pants and shirt back on and walked out of the dressing room.

He smiled and said, "Did you like them?"

I looked at him and softly said, "None of them fit. They were too tight."

Good husband that he was, he just cheerfully said, "Well, maybe we should try some of those clothes over there." He pointed at the plus-size section.

If I used bad language, I would have used it then. Instead, I just whispered, "Okay."

Together we selected some of the less ugly outfits, and back I went into the dressing room. Through trial and error, I found that I was a size 22/24, and even those clothes were a bit tight. However, I reasoned that I was going to lose the baby weight soon. Then I could donate the ugly pants, long knit shirts, and horrible jumpers to Goodwill. We left the store with the beginnings of a plus-size wardrobe. I also left the store with a feeling I had never experienced before when it came to my appearance: utter misery.

Lost in a Fat Woman's Body

So many times, I wished that day in the mall would have been the tipping point for me—that I would have gotten serious about my weight problem and fixed it. Instead, I kept gaining weight and getting bigger. The three years between Rachel's and Grace's birth brought many joyous times, as well as many embarrassing moments. I resorted to making most of my own clothes, and with every pound I gained, I lost some self-esteem. I stopped volunteering at church, avoided social situations, and sat on the couch as much as I could. My life had become one embarrassing moment after another. One Sunday at church stands out.

During the service, my youngest daughter started to get fussy. I took her out through the back of the auditorium and waddled slowly down the hall to the nursing room. I reached the small room that was set aside for mothers and babies. It had a changing table, a restroom, and several rocking chairs arranged in a circle. When I opened the door, I saw four or five of my friends sitting in the room with their babies. I walked in, sat down in one of the chairs, and enjoyed conversation with the other mothers while I rocked Grace. I tried not to compare my squishy stomach with their slim and trim figures, but I had a hard time keeping my eyes off their lack of fat. I was starting to feel like I needed some Oreos.

When I realized the service was almost over, I began to get up out of the chair, but when I stood up, the chair came with me. There I was, half-standing, with a rocking chair attached to my butt.

My next move was swift and sure. I quickly lowered the chair back to the ground and sat down. The women in the room were mortified. No one knew where to look, especially me. I was afraid to try standing up again, but I knew I could not spend the rest of the morning in the rocking chair. This time I pushed down hard on the arm of the chair with one hand and held onto Grace with the other hand. With some shifting and tugging, I popped out of the chair and fled the room.

2

I Tried Not to Be Fat

I understood I was fat. Seat belt extenders, plus-size clothing shops, plummeting self-esteem, and the reduced ability to participate in life's joys and challenges were part of my reality. I tried denying how I looked and avoided mirrors at all costs, but photographs do not lie. I tried accepting myself as an obese woman, but I could not do it. Somewhere in my mind, I believed that I should neither weigh 300 pounds nor accept myself as an obese woman.

I remember well the days when cameras didn't provide instant results. You had to take your film to the store, wait seven days, and drive back to the store to pick up your developed pictures. It's not so much the process I recall but sitting in the parking lot of the camera shop, opening the package of pictures, sliding the glossy stack out of the envelope, and then gasping in horror. I would start shuffling through the images like a deck of cards. Children playing—cute. Birthday parties—so much fun. What is that fat blob in the edge of that picture? Me! I would stop and stare. *Who is that woman?*

I knew I was wearing a size 26/28, but sometimes I could not really see what that looked like. I knew the last time I had stepped on the scale it was almost to its 300-pound capacity. But I could not picture what I looked like to other people.

This is why I don't get my picture taken, I would scream at myself. *The camera just isn't kind to me.* I would quickly shuffle through the rest of the pictures, not really enjoying them, because all I could think about was the one picture I was in. *Why did John take my picture?* I would fume internally. *He knows I hate getting my picture taken.*

Before I got home, I would remove the offending pictures and throw them in the trash. If they recorded something important, like my birthday or Mother's Day, I would keep the best ones and ditch the others. That's why if you look at the before pictures in this book, you won't find any posed portraits—no "You look great today. Let me take your picture" shots. Just random pictures that I allowed someone to snap when my defenses were down.

Time after time, I looked at pictures of myself and stared in disbelief. Every single picture surprised me, which says something about my lack of self-perception. Certain pictures, such as this one, were worse than others.

The picture was taken in 1994 for a directory at our church in Tallahassee, Florida. I had lost weight after Grace's birth and was down to about 250 pounds. Soon after this picture was taken, I mistakenly thought I had my diet under control. Instead of continuing to watch my portion sizes and cut back on eating sweets, I fell back into my familiar, unhealthy eating habits. The weight began coming back. When the church offered free portraits to any family that chose to participate in the directory, I temporarily overcame my hatred of photos and decided to sit for the picture. I wanted us to look our best, so I had lovingly smocked matching dresses for the girls. John had a great-looking suit, but I had a problem. As usual, I had nothing to wear. My sunflower jumper with the plastic buttons would not fit. Nor would the green-flowered outfit I had made a few months earlier. I had outgrown that outfit one month after I made it and had thrown it in the trash.

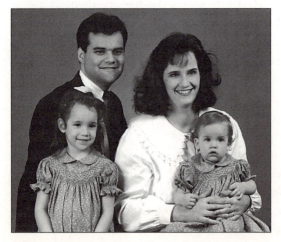

While you may see a smiling woman with curly hair, all I could see was the beginning of a double chin, huge arms, and fat hands.

The day before we were scheduled to get tortured by the photographer, I stood in my closet feeling angry and frustrated. Flipping through the few clothes that fit, I spied a long black skirt. The floor-length skirt had been part of my outfit for a church musical the year before. I had to make the skirt, because I was too fat to wear the outfit my choir director had ordered for the other women. I remember being humiliated that my skirt was different from everyone else's and relieved when he put me in the back row.

I pulled the skirt out of my closet and held it in front of me. I hoped it still fit. Stepping into the skirt, I began to pull it up over my thighs, but it got stuck mid-thigh. So I did the next best thing and put it up and over my head. To my relief, it was not tight around my hips. Nor should it have been, since I had used almost 9 yards of fabric! However, I could not get the waistband to close. What to do now? Well, there was always the rubber band trick, where you give yourself a little bit of stretch by looping a rubber band through the buttonhole and sliding the button through the loop. On the other hand, I could alter the skirt or just not tuck in the blouse. I eventually added a little piece of fabric onto the end of the waistband and had my picture taken.

The next week we went back to the church to see our pictures and to order prints for family and friends. The salesperson reached her hand into the white envelope, pulled out an 11 x 14, and set it on her display easel. I was shocked. John looked great, Rachel was beautiful, Grace was adorable, and I was fat. I could not believe my eyes. Who was that women with the double chin, the wide shoulders, and the chest that looked like it belonged on someone else? I looked at that lady and then at John and said, "No thank you. We won't be ordering any of those pictures." She was very gracious and gave us our free 8 x 10. I took that picture, stuck it in a box, and put the lid on it.

I Tried to Change

Even though I had a hard time picturing what I looked like to other people, I knew I needed to lose weight. I only needed to see my thighs hanging off the sides of a chair or feel my embarrassment when walking into a room to remember how fat I had become.

I was a constant dieter. Dieting was a pastime, a hobby, a waste of money, and a continual source of frustration. Over and over I would join a program, commit to a new eating plan, or promise myself I would change. I never followed through on any of my promises and was always frustrated with myself. But I did not give up. I'd see an advertisement for Weight Watchers on television, and off I'd trot to join once again. If I wasn't on Weight Watchers, I was trying another diet plan, one I had seen on television or read about in a magazine or book. You'd think I would just quit wasting my money, but the desire to lose weight and make a permanent change burned within me.

Weight Watchers

I joined Weight Watchers so many times that I should have had my own parking space in front of the building. I was like a yo-yo. Join, try for a week, quit for two. Join, try for two weeks, quit for three. Over and over again, I gave Weight Watchers a try. Weight Watchers is a great program if you follow its plan. If you ignore the advice, you won't lose weight. I was very good at ignoring the advice.

Weight Watchers is one of the oldest surviving weight-loss programs in the country and has helped millions of people lose weight. The program, started by Jean Nidetch, works by assigning point values to all the foods you consume. If you eat within your points and exercise regularly, you can be successful on the plan. The first time I joined Weight Watchers was before I had become medically obese. It was just after our Georgia trip, and I was tired of tight suits, unflattering jeans, and freaking out when I stood on the scale. That Weight Watchers experience went well for me. I lost 20 pounds in just a couple of months and felt better than I had since before I got married. But I did not reach my goal weight and quit before going through the six-week maintenance program. Predictably, I gained the 20 pounds back and added several more. Needless to say, I was mad at myself. Why did I gain all that weight back after working so hard to lose it? Why couldn't I keep my weight down to a level that made me happy? I couldn't seem to admit that eating junk day after day and never exercising had anything to do with it. I was not ready to take responsibility for the problem.

As my weight went from bad to worse, I still tried losing with Weight Watchers. Over a period of several months, I rejoined at least five times. Weight Watchers has a great plan. You do not have to pay thousands of dollars upfront as with some other weight-loss centers. You do not have to buy their food. You just have to show up each week and get weighed. If you miss a week, it's okay. But you do have to pay for the week you missed. It's ingenious really—a great financial incentive to keep coming. But I would attend for a few weeks and then miss a couple, because I had eaten like a pig. When I'd show up again at the check-in table, the staff would explain that it would be less expensive for me to just rejoin rather than pay for the weeks I had missed. So I would start over with a fresh folder, determined to make it work.

But I was not ready to make it work. For example, I normally attended Saturday morning meetings. I quickly figured out that if I ate very little on Friday, I could probably weigh a few ounces less on Saturday morning. I would wear the lightest clothes I could get away with. Sometimes I even put potential outfits on the scale at home to find the lightest one. At this point, I weighed well above 250 pounds, so what possible difference did the weight of a shirt make? Nonetheless, once I had eaten sparingly on Friday and picked out the lightest outfit for the Saturday morning meeting, off I went. I would stand on the scale and just pray: *Dear God, please let me have lost 1 pound.* Sometimes my deceit was rewarded. The Weight Watchers employee would say, "You did great this week. You lost a half pound." I would take my little folder and sit on the too-small metal folding chair, hoping my backside did not infringe on the person next to me, and prepare myself for the meeting. The meetings were always informative, but I listened with only one ear, as my mind busily thought about my next meal.

By the time the meeting adjourned, I had convinced myself it would be okay to drive through my friendly fast-food restaurant, which just happened to be right down the road. After all, I would not have to weigh in again for a whole week. I would waddle out to my car, get in, and drive directly to McDonald's, where I would happily order two sausage biscuits, two orders of hash browns, one coffee, and one diet drink. (I ordered two beverages so the McDonald's employee would not think I was going to eat all the food myself.) My week would go by in much the same way. I would alternate healthy choices and small portions with extremely large amounts of high-fat, high-sugar foods. Before long I quit going to the weigh-ins, quit trying to make healthy choices, and fell right back into my old habits 24/7. Repeatedly, Weight Watchers and I joined forces, and although Weight Watchers kept its end of the bargain, I never kept mine.

Fad Diets

As part of my never-ending quest to lose weight, I often tried fad diets featured in magazines and books. I did avoid extreme diets that I knew to be unhealthy, such as those that recommended using supplements or protein drinks to lose weight quickly. However, as an avid reader, I always found the newest diet book to be irresistible. The wonderful pictures of thin people on the front cover, and the promise of a changed life, had me handing money to the bookstore cashier on a regular basis. I would devour each book, loving every minute of it, committing to following its advice. Inevitably, I failed to keep the promise to myself.

I read books and magazine articles about diets that promoted one food group over another or promised that a certain way of eating increased metabolism and burned fat effectively. One magazine diet had me eating boiled eggs, pickles, and cottage cheese with every meal. I managed to stick with that awful diet for about seven days and actually lost 5 pounds, but once I quit eating that disgusting combination of foods every day, I gained all the weight back, plus 3 more pounds. It was all quite depressing.

Sometimes I dieted by counting calories religiously (for about five days) or exclusively eating frozen diet dinners for both lunch and dinner. I avoided sugar, attempted to drink ten glasses of water a day, and bought low-calorie foods for weeks at a time. No matter what I tried, I never lost much weight. Even though I temporarily changed some of my eating habits while I was trying diet after diet, I never completely gave up eating large quantities of high-fat foods. The healthy diets such as Weight Watchers would have worked if I had done a better job in following their plans, while the fad diets, such as eating strange combinations of foods, would never have resulted in sustained weight loss.

I was very susceptible to huge headlines on magazine covers. The words, "I lost 50 pounds in 6 weeks and still ate anything I wanted" appealed to me. I desperately wanted to believe those promises. Even though in the back of my mind I knew these claims had to be hoaxes, I was happy to suspend disbelief long enough to buy the magazine and take it home. I knew it had taken me longer than six weeks to gain 50 pounds, so it just made sense it was going to take longer than six weeks to lose 50 pounds. Even so, once I got home, I would tear out the pages showing amazing before and after pictures and tape them inside my closet door. Every time I reached into my closet for yet another ugly jumper, I saw the pictures and became reinvigorated. Well, at least for as long as it took me to walk back into the kitchen. Later on, I would pore over the recipes provided and vow to try that particular diet. Sometimes I even made a special trip to the grocery store to make sure I had all the right ingredients. At the grocery store, I would also replenish my chocolate stash for those times when the diet got hard. Predictably, I did not lose much weight, if any.

"As Seen on TV"

Although I never used any kind of diet supplements, I loved to watch the infomercials on television late at night. I resisted all the programs, except for Richard Simmons's Deal-A-Meal. The $99 price tag was steep for us, but you could make "three easy payments of just $33." After joining Weight Watchers so many times, $99 seemed like a bargain. I picked up the phone late one night and placed my order.

A few days later, a little box arrived in the mail. It was full of interesting folders, brightly colored cards, and an exercise video or two. How fun! How exciting! How did it all work? I never found out. I read the information, moved the cards around inside the folders, stuck the box in a drawer, and eventually sold the system at a yard sale for $3. The plan was probably fine, but I'll never be able to tell you for sure, because I never even gave it a chance.

That Little Thing Called Hope

You would think that after trying to lose weight for ten years, I would have given up—especially since I was actually gaining weight on a monthly basis. Even so, somewhere inside I never completely gave up hope that I would be able to lose weight. Privately, where no one could see, I longed to make a change. I cried sometimes, out of frustration and out of sadness over what I had allowed myself to become. Somewhere in that secret place, I still had hope.

What are your secret hopes for yourself? Part of moving forward to a new phase of life is acknowledging where you have come from. To that end, let's look at your history with diets.

Your Turn

Have you tried to lose weight before? .... Yes ❏ No ❏

What types of diets have you tried and what were the results? Be detailed and specific. _____

_____

_____

Diet Results

How does it feel to see in writing some of the different plans, programs, and attempts you have made to lose weight? For me it served as a stark reminder of the time, money, and energy I had invested over the years with no long-term results. It made me feel like a failure and a loser.

Feelings Past and Present

As you journey down this road with me, be honest with yourself concerning food, your appearance, and your goals. The emotional side of weight loss is often the hardest battle to win. One dear friend used to tell me, "Diane, I don't have an emotional attachment to food. I just love to eat!" But after years and years of saying that, she finally confessed, "Well, maybe I do have some emotional issues with food." That admission was the turning point for her. Regardless of where you are right now, being honest about your feelings will move you one step closer to achieving the goals you have set for yourself.

I often think about how I felt as a fat person. I felt ugly. I felt unworthy. I felt like a failure. Moreover, I often felt that people looked at me with scorn and disdain. Being overweight is a public problem. We cannot hide our size from the world. People who struggle with alcohol or other addictive substances are often able to conceal their weaknesses from others, at least for a while. However, when we do not fit into seats comfortably, or take up more space in an elevator than we should, or stop doing something we enjoy because of our size, others know. Sometimes they feel free to comment on it.

Your Turn

When you are in a group, do you ever feel inferior
because of your weight and appearance?.................................Yes ❑ No ❑

If yes, describe a particular situation and how it made you feel: _____
_____

Have you ever been treated differently than others
because of your weight?...Yes ❑ No ❑

Explain what happened. Looking back, were you really treated differently
or was that just your perception? _____
_____
_____

Treatment of the Overweight

In restaurants, I sometimes overheard people making comments about my size. Granted, I was loading up at the buffet table, but the comments still hurt my feelings. Once at a family-style buffet restaurant, a child at the table next to ours said, "Mommy, look how fat that lady is!" I could not help but look at the mom as she told her child to lower her voice. The woman and I locked eyes, and I felt ashamed. Sometimes family members said, "I don't know why you insist on not wearing a coat when it is so cold out." What they knew, but pretended not to, was that I could not find a coat big enough to fit me.

Once in line at Walmart, I heard a child again say, "Look at that fat lady, Mommy." I turned to look and realized with much horror that I was the fat lady. I quickly turned back around and pretended I did not hear her. I listened carefully to her mother's response. To my surprise she just said, "Yes, I see her, but you must speak more quietly in the store." Okay, now the mom was calling me fat too. I didn't know what to do or where to look, so I just stood like a cow waiting for its food. I wanted to sink into the floor in embarrassment, but of course I couldn't. I remained standing there, trying not to cry.

I knew I was heavy, but other people couldn't say it—just me. I could joke about my weight with John and my friends, but they were not allowed to say anything. I told jolly fat people jokes, laughed at other fat jokes, and pretended my weight did not bother me, but it did. I hated walking into a room, realizing that I was waddling as if I were in my third trimester of pregnancy. I abhorred doctor visits and completely avoided the dentist. Sitting in chairs could be embarrassing, and restaurant booths were just too small. But other people had to be quiet about all that. Looking back, I realize that I often made jokes about myself in an attempt to make other people comfortable with my weight or to acknowledge my weight before anyone else could comment. I wish I had been strong enough not to make fun of myself and to stand up to people who made derogatory comments about my appearance.

Unless you have dealt with obvious obesity, you might find it hard to believe how insensitive people can be. Most people would not dare comment on a physical deformity or a mental handicap, but fat comments are allowed and laughed at. That mother in Walmart could have used her daughter's innocent exclamation as a teachable moment, where she explained to her that it is wrong to judge a person based on what they look like or what they wear. Given the mother's response, I wouldn't be surprised if she told her friends what had happened and laughed about it.

I eventually developed a thicker skin and learned to shrink into my own shell when I overheard a rude comment, but each one still hurt. I could excuse the comments young kids made, but comments from adults didn't roll off my shoulders so easily. I hope that as time goes by, we will be more understanding of people with weight problems. When I see overweight people now, I feel extreme empathy and a desire to help. As you travel your own personal road to better health, I hope you will continue to feel empathy for those who struggle with weight while at the same time encouraging them to walk a healthier path.

Sitting on the Sidelines of Life

As hard as it was to hear snide, rude comments, it was even harder to watch life from the sidelines. The more weight I carried, the less I moved. When my weight first went above 250 pounds, I was pregnant with Rachel. I blamed my fatigue and lack of energy on the pregnancy. However, once I recovered from her birth, I no longer had an excuse. Instead of moving my body to get more energy, I sat.

The older Rachel got, the more activities she participated in, and the more tired I became. It took all the energy I had just to get ready for her weekly ballet class. Once there, I would sit on the uncomfortable bench, talking with the others moms, admiring their energy. I could not imagine being involved in as many activities as they were. I was exhausted just walking up the steps to the ballet studio.

Once Grace was born, my energy level decreased even further. And so did my desire to participate in normal day-to-day activities. If a group of moms was planning a trip to the park, I'd reluctantly agree to go, all the while trying to think of an excuse to decline. If I did end up meeting them at the park, I would feel conspicuous waddling around in the sand, trying to keep up with the girls. I would often invent a reason to leave early. I felt so bad for the girls that I'd swing us through Wendy's for a milkshake treat. That made them happier about leaving their friends, and it made me feel better too—at least temporarily. Once again, I used food as a comfort and a solace.

Repeatedly sitting on the sidelines leads to a long list of regrets. I have many regrets, including missing out on the fun of swimming with my daughters. When I began my trip up the scale, I stopped wearing bathing suits, opting for capri pants and a big shirt instead. It was embarrassing to go to a swimming party dressed as if I were meeting friends for lunch. I would stand around on the pool deck, watching other people swim, feeling as conspicuous as an elephant might in your living room. Friends would come visit with me for a short time, but eventually the lure of their children calling, "Mommy come play with me," would take them away from me and back to their fun.

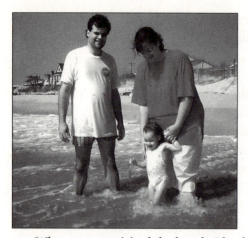

My homemade white capris were soaking wet by the time we finished playing in the water. I remembered wringing them out in the bathroom sink hoping they would dry quickly, as they were the only pants that fit me.

Whenever we visited the beach, I broke out the capris again, suffering through the indignity and discomfort of getting my pants and shirt wet but forcing myself to smile. Although getting messy with sand is fun in a bathing suit, it's not so much fun in capri pants. John would tell me, "Just wear a bathing suit. Who cares?" I would shake my head, refusing to even be drawn into that conversation. I never shared my feelings with John or anyone else. I kept it all inside. I didn't want to admit to John that I was struggling with low self-esteem and feelings of inadequacy. Looking back, I realize he knew there was a problem, and he tried to make me feel better. Nevertheless, there were times when even he got frustrated by my avoidance of certain situations.

When it was time for John's annual office party, I did everything in my power to avoid going. What would people think of me? Would they be able to tell that I had gained weight since the year before? When John mentioned the office party, I often said, "I can't go to the party because I don't have anything to wear." He would then say, "Let's go buy you a new dress." I would resist, he would insist, and we would go on another fruitless shopping trip.

Once I got fat, I hated shopping for myself. It wasn't fun to look for clothes. I was embarrassed to go into Catherine's Stout Shoppe, walk through the doors of Lane Bryant, or even browse in the plus-size section of department stores. When I was in the regular-size section, shopping for a gift, I made a point to say loudly, "Do you think your mom would like this, John?" announcing to the clerks and anyone else in earshot that I was indeed conscious of the size of clothing on the racks. This was to avoid the embarrassment of having a salesclerk politely point me to the plus-size section—an incident that had happened before and that I was bound and determined to never let happen again.

Shopping was hard on my legs and knees too. If the trip began at ten in the morning, by eleven I was exhausted and needed to go home, or at least needed a Cinnabon for short-term energy. My legs ached after only a short amount of walking. I would say, "I'm just not feeling very well. I think I need to go home." Frustrated, John and the kids would look at me and say, "We just got here!" I was in my late twenties, but I felt so tired and old. So I began to avoid shopping trips. I was not above faking a foot injury if someone asked me to do something that required a lot of walking.

Your Turn

Complete these statements:

One time I wanted to _____
_____, *but I stopped myself because of my weight.*

This made me feel _____.

How is your energy level compared to five years ago?
_____
_____

Do you think it could be better?.. Yes ❑ No ❑

Does your lifestyle reflect your abilities and ambitions?......... Yes ❑ No ❑

Does your weight limit your ambitions?................................. Yes ❑ No ❑

The Importance of Believing

My low energy level thwarted my desires, and I struggled daily with this disconnect for the three years I was overweight and the seven years I was obese. Sure, I kept up with my housework and shopped for the children, but the many things I avoided still haunt me. My limited energy meant I had little desire to reach my goals. I missed countless opportunities to participate more actively in my family's life, and I still regret that my weight held me back.

I allowed my own unhappiness to dictate the choices I made in life. Instead of trying to overcome my weight problem, I believed losing weight and keeping it off was impossible. I let mean, insensitive things other people said paralyze me. I struggled with feelings of inadequacy. I felt hopeless because I had so much weight to lose. I identified with my image so strongly that I became my fat. I saw myself as forever fat, which became a self-fulfilling prophecy. I had stopped believing in myself.

Your Turn

Give one honest reason why you have not been able to lose weight, maintain the loss, and get healthy? _____

_____

_____

_____

_____

Which obstacle to losing weight do you wish you could remove? _____

_____

_____

_____

_____

Do you believe in yourself?..Yes ❑ No ❑

List every weight-loss obstacle you can think of, even if you have not personally experienced it. _____

_____

_____

_____

_____

Do you believe it is possible for you to lose weight
and become healthier? .... Yes ❑ No ❑

Overall, do you feel supported by the people in your life? .... Yes ❑ No ❑

How do you know? _____

_____

_____

_____

The Main Weight-Loss Obstacle

Now we come to the crux of the problem. Most of us unconsciously create any number of obstacles and place them directly on our path to weight loss. To discover your own obstacles, look at your excuses. One of my biggest excuses was the number of pounds I needed to lose. When I needed to lose only 20 or 30 pounds, I believed I could lose weight. However, as the years went on and my weight ballooned, I felt the amount I needed to lose was just too great. I also created excuses for why I could not lose weight: It was the wrong time of year because a holiday was on the horizon. Company was coming. I was a busy mother. We were going on vacation. Look back at your answers to the above questions. Did you list *yourself* as a weight-loss obstacle? Are you standing in your own way? I know I was.

The Turning Point

Such was my life as an obese person. I did not become a stronger person when I endured the stares of friends and strangers. Instead, I became a weaker person. Morbid obesity had worn down my dream of losing weight, and I had given up. I was tired of trying. So there I was, sitting in the doctor's office dealing with the cold reality that I had ruined my life. It was 1997, and I had been dealing with obesity for ten years.

How much more weight could I possibly gain? Would I reach 325? 350? 400? For the first time in ten years, I understood the severity of my situation. When you weigh more than a professional football player, could crush your best friend if you fell on her, and can't fit into airplane seats, something is wrong.

When the doctor very gently told me, once again, that I should try to lose weight, I thought to myself, *I can't.* I had tried. For ten years I had tried every diet plan known to man and none had worked.

Even though I did not think I could do it, I was scared enough this time to try again. My blood pressure was starting to elevate, and my cholesterol levels were no good either. My knees hurt, and I was often out of breath. I was worried about my health.

Frankly, I also worried about clothes. Wearing a size 26/28 put me at the top sizing of plus-size departments. I could not imagine where I would find clothes if I continued to gain weight. As I walked out of the office that day, I felt like a two-ton truck. I remember sitting in the car with my head on the steering wheel, crying out of frustration. "What is wrong with me? Why am I so fat?"

3

Preparing for Your Journey

Now that you have examined some of your personal weight-loss attempts and the obstacles that stand in your way, let's take another step forward and prepare for success.

I regret not doing two things before I started to lose weight. First, I regret not taking a formal "before" picture. It is important as you begin your weight-loss journey to document where you start. A "before" photo will let you see how far you have come and will encourage you when the inevitable weight-loss plateaus occur.

I also regret not taking detailed measurements of my body. When I first began losing weight, I took only my waist and hip measurements. Once I had recorded those, my depression was overwhelming. I do not know if my self-esteem could have taken the added toll of recording the girth of my thighs, calves, arms, and neck. Regardless of how disheartening it may be, I advise you to endure the discomfort and measure everything you can. As you lose weight, your entire body will change—not just your waist and hips. There were times when I lost only a fraction of a pound, but my clothes felt a little looser than they had the week before. By taking my measurements early on, I had a tangible way to mark my progress without worrying about the number on the scale. As you do weight training and cardiovascular workouts, you will build lean muscle mass and burn fat. Your body measurements will help you see that change as it occurs.

Your Turn

Look in the mirror with a minimal amount of clothes on. Be perfectly frank with yourself. How do you look? How do you feel when you look in the mirror? _____

_____

_____

_____

_____

Take your measurements and write them down.
Waist: _____
Hips: _____
Chest: _____
Upper arms: _____
Upper thighs: _____
Wrist: _____
Calves: _____

Do you have a current picture of yourself? If not, take one now.

The Tape Measure Was Too Short

When I finally got up the courage to measure my waist and hips, it was a frightening experience. I hadn't measured myself since I was first married. I still remember standing in my bedroom, tape measure in hand. I sucked in my breath and gingerly put the soft fabric of the yellow tape measure around my waist. Because my waist stuck out farther than my chest, it was easy to read the number: 55.5 inches. I sucked in my breath harder and pulled the tape measure a little bit tighter. That was better: 55 inches was the new, official measurement. I remember thinking about that number for a little bit and realizing that 55 inches was Rachel's height at seven years old. I wanted to stop right there and cry, but I pushed forward and tried to measure my hips. I say "tried," because my tape measure was only 60 inches long and my hips were bigger than that. *Okay*, I thought to myself, *how awful that this tape measure is too short to measure my hips.*

Notice that I was annoyed at the tape measure's length and not at myself for the size of my hips. Being a seamstress, I found the solution to the tape measure problem. I grabbed some string, wrapped it around my hips, and then measured the string: 65 inches. I was as big around as my best friend, Jane, was tall. That was a sobering thought, and one that upset me so much that I almost went off on a binge.

Instead of bingeing on food, I stood in my bedroom and had a heart-to-heart conversation with myself. I went over the reasons I wanted to lose weight, I recalled how scared I had been while standing on the scale at the doctor's office, and I looked in my closet to see all the ugly clothes hanging there. I knew then that the last thing I wanted to do was quit before I even gave myself a chance to get started. I put the bingeing thought out of my head, gathered up the three children, and went outside. I still remember sitting on my front steps holding little Mark. The girls were joyously riding their bikes up and down the driveway. I sat watching them. More than anything, I wanted to be free from all the fat I'd been lugging around. As much as my waist and hip measurements scared me, the thought of missing out on the rest of my life scared me more.

If you skipped the last set of questions, I encourage you to get a tape measure and just start measuring. Do not worry about what the numbers are right now. In fact, do not even think about them, because you are working on changing your body. Just measure and record. As your body changes, the numbers will change as well. Today my waist measures 28 inches and my hips 38 inches. I am satisfied with those numbers (especially after giving birth to seven children). In fact, I no longer think in terms of numbers but only in terms of how good I feel and how full my life is.

Your Turn

Can you picture yourself as a fit, thin person? .... Yes ❏ No ❏

How does it feel when you imagine being at your desired size and fitness level? _____

_____

_____

Do you believe you can finally be successful? .... Yes ❑ No ❑

Why or why not? _____

_____

_____

Goal Setting

It may not be easy, but visualize yourself at the size you want to be. I had been fat for so long that I could not even imagine how I would look at a lower weight. The fat Diane had been part of me for a decade, and I was not convinced that the thin Diane was still inside. One thing that helped me was taping an old picture of my thin self to the refrigerator. Every time I walked past the refrigerator, the image strengthened my resolve. I had been thin and fit. I could be that way again.

Becoming thin and fit was just one of my goals in losing weight. What was the first thing that entered your mind when I mentioned the word *goals*? Did you automatically think of a goal in terms of weight or size? Or did you think of a goal in terms of an activity level, a health issue, or something else?

As you can imagine, I had many weight-loss goals during my years of obesity. Being on a diet more often than not, I was always trying to attain a particular number on the scale. But instead of moving closer to my desired weight, I kept moving farther and farther away from it. I failed miserably at every diet I tried, and with each failure I gained more weight. This last time, I chose to look at my life as a whole, not just as a number. Instead of focusing on the scale, I set some very specific goals for myself.

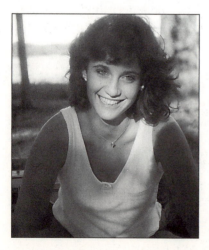

This picture was taken shortly before John and I were married. I loved how I could see my collarbones and cheekbones.

Your Turn

Have you had a weight-loss goal in the past?..........................Yes ❏ No ❏

What was your goal based on (check all that apply)?
❏ Size   ❏ Inches lost
❏ Number on the scale   ❏ Other _____

Did you achieve your goal?...Yes ❏ No ❏

What are your current weight-loss goals (check all that apply)?

❏ Pounds lost (provide   ❏ Self-confidence
   number) _____   ❏ Appearance
❏ Clothing size   ❏ Lifestyle
❏ Body measurements/inches lost ❏ Look good for upcoming event
❏ Blood pressure or other health ❏ Fitness level
   measurement   ❏ Healthy eating habits
❏ Energy level   ❏ Bad habit elimination
❏ Self-perception   ❏ Other _____

Notice that this list of goals is not related only to how much you weigh but also to other important aspects of life. Your goals can and should be both tangible and intangible.

Set Goals, Get Focused and Take Action

Goal setting is a vital part of our lives. We live in a society that encourages us to reach for something more. How do we do that? We determine a goal based on things such as desires, family expectations, societal pressures, or a perception that life will be different when we make a change, acquire something, or lose something. Once we identify what it is we want (or don't want), we take action.

For me, the action part was easier said than done. I had always found it easy to pick a goal but very difficult to follow through. I found it hard to reach my goals because they seemed too big—150 pounds was too much to focus on without getting overwhelmed. So this time, to stay focused, encourage action, and avoid the frustration I had felt in the past, I did several things:

- Broke my huge weight-loss goal into 5-pound increments
- Set small weekly goals that weren't scale related
- Worked on one habit at a time instead of trying to change everything at once
- Recommitted to my goals daily
- Shared my goals with my husband
- Wrote down my goals

Your Turn

Look over the list of goals on page 35. What goal besides losing weight speaks to you the most? I encourage you to work on that goal this week.

My goal this week is: _____

_____

_____

_____

To achieve that goal, I will commit to: _____

_____

_____

_____

_____

Write down your long-term goals and put your list where you will see it every day, such as on the refrigerator. Or tape it in your desk drawer, where you will notice it every time you reach for a pen. Wherever you put it, remember it. Pull out your list, look at it, and take time to evaluate where you are. As you start reaching your goals, it's important to reassess them, because you will most likely identify even more opportunities for success than you first imagined.

Afraid to Fail

As you work through developing some concrete goals, you might find yourself feeling fearful. I did. I was almost afraid to try again, because I was afraid I would once again fail. I was almost afraid to succeed because I couldn't imagine how sweet life would be once I had conquered my obsession with food. Fear of failure is real.

It's not fun or easy to admit that you've failed. It's hard to look your husband in the eye and confess that you ate all the cookies in the pantry. It's uncomfortable to admit that you no longer fit into regular-size clothes. And for me, it was hard to confess that I had failed at yet another diet.

When I made the decision to try to lose weight one more time, I had a lot of fear. I was afraid I would fail. But within that fear sat a kernel of hope—the hope that this time would be different and I would finally get it right.

As you read this book and examine some of your motivations, perceptions, and obstacles, my wish is that you find the hope you need to put failure behind you and that you begin to have success with weight loss.

Your Turn

Do you think fear has any part in the failure or success
of weight loss? .... Yes ❑ No ❑

Explain why you feel the way you do: _____

_____

_____

What fears do you have concerning food, dieting, and exercise? _____

_____

Does fear of failure stop you from trying to get healthy? ...... Yes ❑ No ❑

Why or why not? _____

_____

_____

In setting your goals and working through any fear of failure, understand that no matter how much weight you need to lose, the emotions are the same. When I was 30 pounds overweight, I felt the same mental anguish and fear as when I was 100 pounds overweight. Even if you want to lose only 10 pounds, your 10 pounds is just as important to you as my 150 pounds was to me.

Three Tips to Get You Started

I approached my weight loss in three major ways. These tips might sound simple, but they were some important keys to my success. These tips, along with the personal goals you have listed in previous questions, should help get your mind going in the right direction.

Share Selectively

I used to share all my weight-loss attempts with any friend or family member who would listen. This time I told just my husband and my closest friend. I kept my effort private because I was afraid I wouldn't succeed. Keeping the journey private has many benefits. It makes the journey sacred. It conserves energy for the real work of losing weight. And, perhaps most importantly, it encourages you to take ownership of your weight and your journey. It becomes your job, your project—one that you've committed to out of respect for yourself, not because you need to prove to others that you are trying to lose weight or because you want to tell the world that you are once again trying to get healthy.

Select one, two, or three people who love you, and who will be encouraging and positive about your successes, to share your goal with.

Clean Out Your Pantry

The second thing I did was to rid my pantry of unhealthy food and to stop replacing it. In my fat world, I would find all sorts of excuses to buy Oreos, mint chocolate chip ice cream, or chips. I could always fabricate a reason to purchase that wonderful yellow bag of Peanut M&M's. Changing my buying habits wasn't easy, because purchasing high-fat, high-sugar foods was fun. I thoroughly enjoyed standing in the aisle at the store and deciding what treat I wanted. Making the conscious choice not to buy

Misery Loves Company

When choosing your support team, beware. Do not automatically assume that your best friend is the appropriate choice. My best friend turned out to be the best person to share my struggles with, but not the best person to share my successes with.

Jane and I had been friends since we were both young married women. We always shared the ups and downs of married life and life with children. She watched me balloon up from an average size to a morbidly obese woman in a matter of three years. She was there when I tried every diet known to man and failed miserably at each one. She was also there when I finally started losing weight using what I now call my Fit to the Finish plan.

In preparation for my attempt at changing my life, I had rid the house of unhealthy foods, planned my exercise program, and practiced eating proper portions. Every day, I looked at my thin inspiration picture on the refrigerator for encouragement.

One day Jane commented on the picture. "You don't really think you can be that thin again, do you?"

I looked at her and said, "Well, I'm sure going to try." She made a face and went on with her previous conversation. I thought about her comment the rest of the day. I wondered what her motives were. I eventually decided that she didn't mean anything by it, and I went on with the process of losing weight.

Before long, I had lost 50 pounds. The difference in my appearance was minimal. But after losing 100 pounds, the difference was startling to people who hadn't seen me in a while. Everywhere I went, people would embarrass me with their effusive comments. One time before a church service, after I had lost about 60 or 70 pounds, a woman I barely knew grabbed my arm and said, "You look like a different person. How did you do it?" I just told her thank-you and said she could call me later if she wanted to talk.

Because Jane and I were best friends, she was often present when people practically fell over themselves complimenting me. She could not get away from the reality of how my appearance was changing.

When other people complimented me in front of Jane, she stood silent and unsmiling. I do not ever remember her chiming in and saying that she thought I was looking better and more attractive.

As I got thinner and fitter, Jane's comments became more pointed and mean-spirited. I felt such confusion. We had been friends for so long. Why wasn't she happy for me? I chose to share my most important struggles with her, and she wasn't being supportive. It just didn't seem fair.

In the past, I might have let her obvious unhappiness and irritation with my weight loss and bodily changes throw me off track. I probably would have turned to food when I felt hurt by her comments. This time I was strong enough to realize that the problem was hers, not mine. I didn't let her personal issues cloud my goals and objectives, and in some ways her attitude made me a stronger person.

When I finally lost the 150 pounds, Jane was the one person who never said, "Good job." It was hurtful and painful, and even though we struggled on with our friendship for several more years, we eventually drifted apart. That experience taught me a lesson. Don't assume that your friends will be happy for you as you change your lifestyle and get healthy. Looking back, I suppose she was jealous, although she was a normal size herself. Perhaps she liked the fat Diane better than the thin Diane. Perhaps she liked feeling somehow superior to the fat Diane. I share this story to make you aware that some people might not be comfortable with a new and different you. I was the same person I had always been inside, but with some added self-confidence.

So as you choose your support team, choose carefully. I hope you have only supportive friends and family, but even if you do not, you can still be successful at winning the battle with your weight.

those foods was hard. Sometimes I would slip up and find a danger food in my cart. Rather than making an excuse about why I needed chocolate, I would put it back on the shelf or hand it to the cashier, saying I had changed my mind. Sometimes I wanted to snatch the food right back out of her hands, but every time I left the store with healthy food in my cart, I felt triumphant—a feeling I soon came to enjoy more than the rush I got when picking out treats for myself.

Pledge to Exercise

The third thing I did was commit to an exercise program. This was a 180-degree turnaround for me, because I had avoided exercise or physical activity of any type for ten years. I felt a combination of nervousness and excitement. On the one hand, I was nervous because I was not sure I was capable of exercising. After all, just walking through the mall exhausted me. But I was excited when I thought about being able to walk without feeling my thighs rub together or about not having to sit down in the middle of a party because my legs were too tired to hold me up any longer.

If you have begun an exercise program, good for you! If not, let's commit together that you will get out of your comfort zone, get off the couch, and get moving.

Commitment Time

In this chapter, I have asked you to closely examine your history with dieting, your feelings about your appearance, and the goals you have for yourself. I think it's appropriate to end this chapter with you making a commitment to yourself.

Your Turn

Can you make a ten- to twelve-week commitment to focus
on your weight-loss goals? .... Yes ❑ No ❑

What, if anything, needs to change for you to commit to working on your goals? _____

_____

_____

How will you commit to your goals? _____

_____

_____

Signature: _____

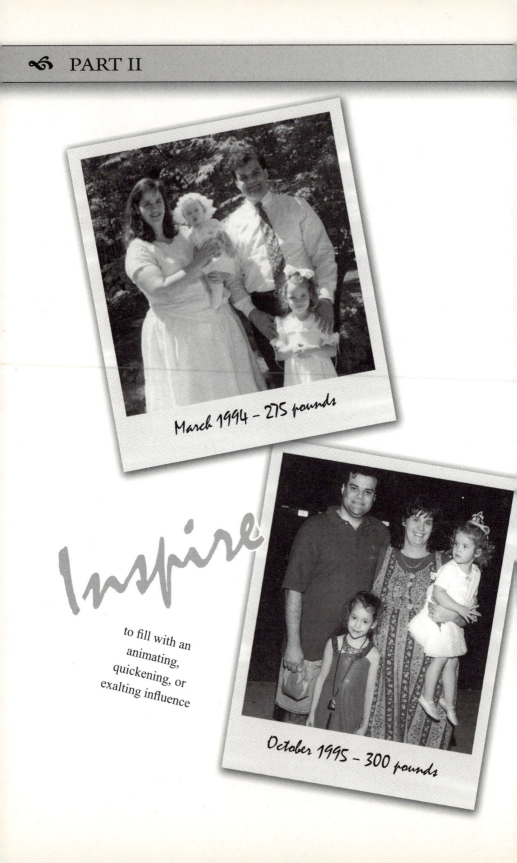

PART II

March 1994 – 275 pounds

Inspire

to fill with an
animating,
quickening, or
exalting influence

October 1995 – 300 pounds

The Fit to the Finish Plan

I never intended to lose weight without the help of an established weight-loss center or health professional, but that is what happened. After I lost my weight, I realized that I had used a plan that other people could also follow to lose weight and keep it off.

With the Fit to the Finish plan, you will learn basic weight-loss principles that you can use now and every day for the rest of your life. In the following chapters, you'll have an opportunity to delve into your personal feelings, thoughts, and emotions surrounding weight and food. As you work through the chapters, you will learn that understanding and acknowledging your emotional relationships to food plays an important role in long-term weight maintenance.

4

The Basics

T hat fateful day in the doctor's office, where I came face to face with my obesity, I realized that I had to change my life. Like you, I made a commitment to myself. I committed to changing my relationship with food and to getting my life back. When I got home from the doctor's office, I did a few things. I measured my hips and waist, pulled out a notebook, and started writing down everything I already knew about dieting and weight loss. If there were a prize for reading diet books and weight-loss articles, I would have won it. I was constantly reading new fitness books, checking dieting books out of the library, and tearing magazine articles out to save for a later time. Like most of you, I knew what to do. This time, I was going to put my knowledge to good use and make a plan tailored for me.

As I wrote down what I knew, I saw a pattern emerge with three recurring themes: be mindful of portion size, avoid unhealthy high-fat foods, and exercise. As I continued to list what I knew about weight loss, things seemed to naturally fall under one of these three categories. I had done it. I knew that I had come up with a plan I was going to follow, even if I hadn't yet given it a name. After I finished analyzing my understanding of weight loss, I had a tangible piece of paper that I could refer back to. I could use that first piece of paper to remind myself that if I quit trying to lose weight, it was not because I did not know how the weight-loss process worked, but rather because I made the choice to ignore what I knew.

Slowly, I began modifying the foods I ate. I stopped nightly binge eating and began taking short walks. From March to the beginning of July

1997, I lost 25 pounds. I started to feel in control of my food choices for the first time since I was a teenager.

I felt as if I were emerging from a cocoon. Even though I was still morbidly obese, I was making positive choices. I started to believe I could actually lose weight and win my life back. I had the clear sense that I was moving forward, never to go back.

Your journey may have taken a lot of twists and turns. No matter how you got to the point where you are today, I applaud you for taking the chance on another weight-loss book. Many books claim to have the perfect solution to weight loss. There is no perfect diet for losing weight. If there were, we would all be fit and healthy. As you begin this chapter, think of Fit to the Finish as a plan, not a diet. Consider it a new way of life that can help you achieve your current weight-loss goals and take you forward for the rest of your life.

When I started losing weight, I knew beyond a shadow of a doubt that I wanted to come up with a sustainable plan. I had lost weight using other programs but had never been able to maintain the weight loss. Why lose weight just to gain it back? In developing my Fit to the Finish plan, I kept that question in the back of my mind. I didn't want to go back into obesity. I wanted to stay fit and healthy. I knew in theory that losing weight shouldn't be that difficult. If I ate fewer calories than I burned, I would lose weight. That's how it should work in a perfect world, but I had a hard time with the eating less part. So I focused first on what I should be eating.

Let's Go

The three major components of the Fit to the Finish plan are fat percentage, portion size, and exercise.

That doesn't seem very complicated, does it? Even though they are simple, each component is equally important; if you ignore one part of the plan, it will be difficult to have long-term success.

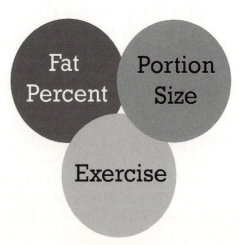

Before delving into each part in detail, let me give you a quick overview of each one.

Percentage of Fat

According to the 2010 *Dietary Guidelines for Americans* from the U.S. Department of Agriculture (USDA), fat should make up between 20 and 35 percent of your diet. The USDA Web site states, "Keep total fat intake between 20 to 35 percent of all calories, with most fats coming from sources of polyunsaturated and monounsaturated fatty acids, such as fish, nuts, and vegetable oils." I chose to eat about 30 percent of my calories from fat, as that seemed like a relatively easy number to adhere to and well within the recommended guidelines.

Portion Size

Portion size is equally important. You hear a lot of people talk about calories, fat grams, and weight lifting, but not many people directly address portion size. If you're a self-described couch potato, you will not lose weight if your portions are geared for a professional football player—it just won't happen.

Exercise

Exercise is vital to both physical and emotional health. Exercise can positively impact your emotions and outlook on life, reducing stress. Your body is designed to move, not to sit in front a computer screen all day or to lie on the couch all night eating potato chips and ice cream. When you are inactive and don't use your body to its full potential, your emotional and physical health suffers.

Moving Forward

In the following three chapters, we will explore your thoughts, ideas, and feelings on fat percentage, portion control, and exercise. Even though you haven't read the entire book yet, start your journey by ridding your pantry of highly processed junk foods, salty chips, or any other food that you instinctively know to be unhealthy for you. Take a few minutes to familiarize yourself with the layout of food labels and pay attention to portion sizes.

5

Percentage of Fat in Your Diet

The truth is, any diet will work if you keep your calories at an appropriate weight-loss level. One weight-loss study, published in the February 2009 *New England Journal of Medicine*, found that the breakdown of participants' food choices mattered less than the fact that they reduced their caloric intake to an appropriate level. But even though you could get away with eating a candy bar for breakfast, lunch, and dinner and still lose weight, you need to keep your overall health in mind. (What's the point of losing weight if you're not going to be healthy enough to enjoy it?)

Keeping my fat consumption around the 30 percent mark enabled me to eat an adequate amount of healthy fats, consume a balanced diet, and even indulge on occasion. To keep it simple, rather than consuming only foods with a 30 percent (or less) fat content, I concentrated on keeping my total fat intake for the day to about 30 percent. The other 70 percent of calories came from whole-grain carbohydrates and lean proteins (more about these later).

Why Fat Percentage?

Why fat percentage and not some other measurement? Well, when I began to get serious about weight loss, I knew I did not want to do any of the following:

- Count calories
- Count fat grams
- Eat special foods

- Abandon favorite family foods
- Give up carbs

- Eat all protein
- Limit my choices
- Deprive myself

That's a big list of what I didn't want. To adhere to the list but still succeed, I needed to try something new. Keeping my intake of fats at about 30 percent made sense to me. It'd be easy to calculate and would provide me with a healthy diet. To this day, I use this method to maintain a healthy weight. I also use this strategy when confronted with an unfamiliar food or when I look back over a day of eating to assess how well I did.

Before you can learn to keep your overall fat consumption to the 30 percent range, you need to learn how to unlock the nutrition labels on the packaged foods you eat. Percentage of fat is not readily apparent on labels, but you can quickly figure out percentage of fat using a pocket or phone calculator. I will show you how to calculate the fat percentage in individual foods, but the important thing to remember is that your fats for the whole day should be in the 30 percent range. This approach will let you cook with healthful oils and even occasionally eat a piece of birthday cake or enjoy a slice of pizza without guilt.

Unlocking the Label

Now that you know that 30 percent is a healthy daily fat intake, it is time to do the math and apply your knowledge in real life. Keeping track of your fat consumption is not rocket science, but you will need to learn a simple formula. Don't be afraid of the word *formula*. It's just third-grade math.

Calories from fat ÷ calories per serving = total % of fat

That is pretty easy, isn't it? To see why you have to calculate the fat percentage in packaged foods, let's look at some actual nutrition labels. You will notice that although labels list many numbers, the percentage of fat is not listed. Calories from fat—yes. Percentage of calories from fat— no. Manufacturers aren't required to list the percentage, and they don't. But don't fear. I'm going to show you how to calculate it, and you may be surprised by what you discover.

Label 1

Label 1 shows both calories per serving and calories from fat.

To determine the fat percentage, simply divide the calories from fat (93) by the total calories per serving (155). Your answer is .60—meaning that 60 percent of the total calories in this food are derived from fat.

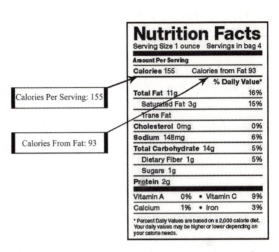

Calories Per Serving: 155

Calories From Fat: 93

Nutrition Facts
Serving Size 1 ounce   Servings in bag 4

Amount Per Serving

Calories 155   Calories from Fat 93

	% Daily Value*
Total Fat 11g	16%
Saturated Fat 3g	15%
Trans Fat	
Cholesterol 0mg	0%
Sodium 148mg	6%
Total Carbohydrate 14g	5%
Dietary Fiber 1g	5%
Sugars 1g	
Protein 2g	

Vitamin A	0%	• Vitamin C	9%
Calcium	1%	• Iron	3%

* Percent Daily Values are based on a 2,000 calorie diet. Your daily values may be higher or lower depending on your calorie needs.

A food such as this, with more than 30 percent of its calories from fat, is not automatically off-limits, because you might also eat lower-fat foods that day. Your goal is to ensure that your total fat percentage for the day stays in line with the recommended fat intake level. So if you have a high-fat snack food such as an avocado (82 percent fat content) for an afternoon snack, pair it with low-fat carrot sticks (3 percent fat content) and pita bread (8 percent fat content) to balance the fat for that snack.

Label 2

The next nutrition label shows that this food has 100 calories per serving and 15 calories from fat.

Using our fat percentage formula, divide calories from fat (15) by calories per serving (100) to get .15. So in this case, 15 percent of the total calories are derived from fat, making this a good food choice.

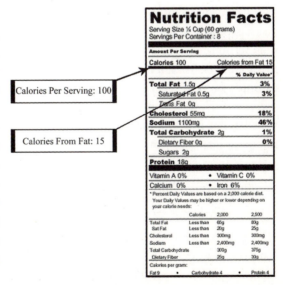

Calories Per Serving: 100

Calories From Fat: 15

Nutrition Facts
Serving Size ¼ Cup (60 grams)
Servings Per Container : 8

Amount Per Serving

Calories 100   Calories from Fat 15

	% Daily Value*
Total Fat 1.5g	3%
Saturated Fat 0.5g	3%
Trans Fat 0g	
Cholesterol 55mg	18%
Sodium 1100mg	46%
Total Carbohydrate 2g	1%
Dietary Fiber 0g	0%
Sugars 2g	
Protein 18g	

Vitamin A 0%	• Vitamin C 0%
Calcium 0%	• Iron 6%

* Percent Daily Values are based on a 2,000 calorie diet. Your Daily Values may be higher or lower depending on your calorie needs:

	Calories	2,000	2,500
Total Fat	Less than	65g	80g
Sat Fat	Less than	20g	25g
Cholesterol	Less than	300mg	300mg
Sodium	Less than	2,400mg	2,400mg
Total Carbohydrate		300g	375g
Dietary Fiber		25g	30g

Calories per gram:
Fat 9   •   Carbohydrate 4   •   Protein 4

Label 3

The third label lists 210 calories per serving with 144 calories from fat.

Again using the formula, calories from fat (144) divided by calories per serving (210) equals .69, or 69 percent of total calories from fat. This food is undoubtedly high in fat, which means you'll need to balance it out with lower-fat foods if you choose to eat it.

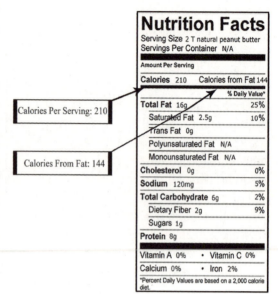

Calories Per Serving: 210

Calories From Fat: 144

Nutrition Facts

Serving Size 2 T natural peanut butter
Servings Per Container N/A

Amount Per Serving

Calories 210   Calories from Fat 144

	% Daily Value*
Total Fat 16g	25%
Saturated Fat 2.5g	10%
Trans Fat 0g	
Polyunsaturated Fat N/A	
Monounsaturated Fat N/A	
Cholesterol 0g	0%
Sodium 120mg	5%
Total Carbohydrate 6g	2%
Dietary Fiber 2g	9%
Sugars 1g	
Protein 8g	

Vitamin A 0%	•	Vitamin C 0%	
Calcium 0%	•	Iron 2%	

*Percent Daily Values are based on a 2,000 calorie diet.

More Practice

Appendix A contains a practice page with ten more fat percentage calculations. After you complete those calculations, practice with a few boxes and cans from your pantry. Once you've done five or six calculations, you will be an expert. If you eat out a lot, do an online search for nutrition information on the meals at your favorite restaurants. You can also download many nutrition-related Smartphone apps, such as the Fast Food Calorie Counter from SparkPeople and the Calorie Counter by FatSecret. Some apps break down the nutritional value of food even further. Others provide detailed information about fast-food and other restaurant meals. You might be surprised how much information is available.

What about Fresh Foods?

Now that you can easily calculate the fat percentage of packaged foods (and some restaurant meals), what do you do for fresh foods, such as vegetables, fish, or meats? The easiest way to determine the amount of fat in fresh foods is via Web sites dedicated to healthy eating, such as SparkPeople (www.sparkpeople.com), FitDay (www.fitday.com), and MyFitnessPal (www.myfitnesspal.com). Simply type in the food you want nutritional information for and apply the fat percentage calculation to the food. Although more complex to negotiate, the USDA's Nutrient Data Laboratory, at www.nal.usda.gov/fnic/foodcomp/search, gives highly detailed information for a wide variety of foods and beverages, including some fast-food options. If you want a calorie reference book for your purse or briefcase, I recommend the *Pocket Calorie Counter* (2011 edition), complied by Suzanne Beilenson.

When following the Fit to the Finish plan, you will balance your fat intake throughout the day, so that about 30 percent of your daily calories are from healthy fats. In the following example, notice that the fat percentages in the foods vary, but the overall total percentage of fat consumed falls at about 30 percent. Also notice that you can have three healthy, filling meals, two snacks, and a fruit cup drizzled with honey for dessert.

Breakfast	*Serving Size*	*Calories*	*Fat Percentage*
Low-fat Greek yogurt	8 oz	137	2.9
Walnuts	.5 oz	93	90
Raspberries	1/4 c	16	less than 1
Black coffee, tea, or water	8 oz	0	0
Totals		**246**	**48**

Lunch	*Serving Size*	*Calories*	*Fat Percentage*
Lentil soup	1 c	210	0
Green salad with Swiss chard	1 c	60	0
Hummus	2 tbsp	50	51
Toasted pita	4-in size	74	less than 1
Totals		**394**	**13**

Snacks	*Serving Size*	*Calories*	*Fat Percentage*
Whole-wheat crackers	8 crackers	157	30
Cheddar cheese	.5 oz	57	74
Raisins	50 raisins	78	less than 1
Apple	1 apple	95	less than 1
Totals		**387**	**24**

Dinner	Serving Size	Calories	Fat Percentage
Roasted cod	6 oz	144	< 1
Leafy green salad	1 1/2 c	40	< 1
Olive oil vinaigrette	1 tbsp	119	100
Feta cheese	.5 oz	37	73
Whole-wheat roll	1 small roll	96	16
Totals		*436*	*38*

Dessert	Serving Size	Calories	Fat Percentage
Fruit cup	1 c	80	< 1
Honey	1 tsp	40	0
Totals		*120*	*<1*
Overall Daily Totals		*1,583*	*30.75*

Source: USDA Nutrient Data Laboratory

Limiting my fat intake was hard at first, because I loved high-fat foods. However, when I started using the fat percentage formula, I realized that the fat in many of my favorite foods was nowhere close to 30 percent. It was usually 50 percent or higher. Below is how my favorites stacked up. I am almost embarrassed to tell you that the average fat percentage in these junk and snack foods is 70 percent.

Food	Serving Size	Calories	Fat Percentage
Oreos	6 cookies	320	38
Chocolate chips	1 c	899	51
Ranch salad dressing	4 tbsp	296	98
Sour cream	3 tbsp	69	91
Homemade biscuit	1 (4-in size)	357	40
Butter	2 tbsp	200	100

I knew I had to change my ways and make better, lower-calorie, lower-fat choices—and change I did! I got rid of unhealthy foods such as chocolate chips and salad dressings by donating unopened packages to a food bank. I make it sound easy, but you almost had to pry the Oreos out of my hand when it was time to actually give the box to a volunteer. Throwing away opened items was hard too, but I'm proud to say that I didn't fish anything out of the garbage. When shopping, I reluctantly put back unhealthy, unnecessary foods that contained more than 30 percent of their calories from fat. For quick calculation when shopping, I developed a pocket chart of common foods and their fat percentages (provided in appendix B). This handy chart prevented me from purchasing items I used to put in my cart on a regular basis.

While pushing your cart through the grocery store, make a concerted effort to select the healthier alternatives to your previous "food friends." Before every grocery store or convenience store trip, I reminded myself of the written commitment I had made. I knew that the purchases I was about to make would either move me toward or away from my goal. I was never sorry when I pulled out of the parking lot with bags full of healthy food in the trunk of my car.

Tools to Help You

See appendix B for a pocket-size chart of fat percentages in common foods. See appendix C for a cheat sheet for calculating fat percentages. You can copy these lists (maybe even have them laminated), stick them in your purse or wallet, and take them to the store with you.

Understanding Marketing Tools

When you look at the front of a food package and see that it declares "No Trans Fat" or "Zero Fat," you might be inclined to purchase it. Before you do, look at the ingredient list to be sure that the food contains healthy, mostly natural ingredients. For example, cereals are made of grains, which have very little fat. But to enhance the flavor of cereals, food manufacturers often add sugar, which does not alter the fat content but does increase sugar and calorie content. Whole-grain cereals with little or no added sugar are healthier choices than cereals with high sugar content.

While you should always read the labels and ingredient lists for the foods you purchase, be especially careful with boxed foods, canned beans, soups, seasoned rice, and sauces. These foods may contain partially hydrogenated vegetable oils, high amounts of sodium (which is essentially salt), chemical preservatives, and saturated fats that you are trying to avoid.

By purchasing low-fat versions of foods, I assumed I would be cutting calories and therefore losing weight. But as I worked through my year of weight loss, I realized that there is often little calorie difference between the low-fat and regular-fat versions of the same foods. Shopping requires diligence and attention to detail. As you plan meals and purchase foods, be sure to examine the labels carefully.

Other Information on the Label

When reading food labels for fat content, you will notice many other numbers. You might be tempted to do what I used to do and ignore them, but as boring or overwhelming as the numbers may seem, they do provide a lot of information beyond fat calories and serving sizes. I would be remiss if I didn't mention some of the other information worth paying attention to, including types of fat, vitamins and minerals, fiber, food additives, and sodium.

A Closer Look at Fats

I've encouraged you to cut back on unhealthy fatty foods, not to eliminate fat entirely. Fats in general get a bad rap, but it's important to realize that there are different types of fats—and some of them are necessary for a healthy diet.

I have to confess, when I was a big girl, the bad fats were the kind of fats I loved. Almost all my favorite foods were highly processed and therefore full of unhealthy fats. Let's look at what types of fats to embrace and what types to avoid.

Unhealthy Fats

Saturated fats and trans fats are two of the big bad fats. They contribute to high cholesterol and can increase your risk of cardiovascular disease. Saturated fats may also increase your chances of developing type 2 diabetes. Whenever you see trans fats or partially hydrogenated oils on a food label, put the item back. Be wary of any foods that contain saturated fats.

Saturated fats: Saturated fats can increase your risk of heart disease and heighten levels of low-density lipid cholesterol ("bad cholesterol"). The American Heart Association (AHA) recommends that the average adult consume no more than 7 percent of his or her daily calories from saturated fats. Foods containing high amounts of saturated fats include animal products such as meat, poultry skin, eggs, fried seafood, dairy products, and butter. Coconut, palm, and other tropical oils contain mostly saturated fats. Research shows that coconut oil may be a healthier choice than vegetable oil. Even so, coconut oil contains about 120 calories per tablespoon, making it a high-calorie addition to your diet.

Trans fats: Trans fats are found naturally in certain animal foods, but the majority of trans fats are created during the manufacturing process, when unsaturated fats undergo partial hydrogenation (adding hydrogen to naturally liquid vegetable oils to make them more solid). Hydrogenation gives foods a longer shelf life, thus increasing the amount of time a product can be stored. In their solid form, trans fats are similar to saturated fats.

Trans fats increase your risk of heart disease. In a perfect world, you would eat no trans fats. However, they can be hard to avoid completely. The AHA recommends eating no more than 1 percent of your calories from trans fats. Note that companies are allowed to list the amount of trans fat in a product as 0 if the product contains less than .5 gram (g) of trans fat per serving. So even if the label says 0, the product might contain some trans fat. To make certain there really is no trans fat, check the ingredient listing. Trans fat will show up as hydrogenated or partially hydrogenated oil. Trans fats are commonly found in packaged foods, in restaurant meals, and in some brands of margarine.

Better Fat Choices

Monounsaturated and polyunsaturated fats are better fat choices than their unhealthier cousins.

Monounsaturated fats: Monounsaturated fats are found in foods such as olive oil, peanut oil, canola oil, avocados, nuts, and seeds. Unlike trans fats and other processed fats, these are naturally occurring fats. Choosing monounsaturated fats over saturated fats does not lower your caloric intake, as all fats have about the same number of calories per serving, but it does offer proven health benefits, including lowering the risk of heart disease and improving blood cholesterol levels.

Government Regulation of Fats

In 2006 the New York Board of Health ruled that by July 2008, all restaurants had to stop including artificially created trans fats in their foods. California passed a similar ban on trans fats in restaurant foods and retail baked goods in 2008. Several major cities in Connecticut and Maryland also ban trans fats. Most cities and states do not have such bans, however, and U.S. obesity rates continue to rise.

While banning trans fats from restaurant foods and retail establishments may be a good step, ultimately the responsibility to eat right lies with the consumer. Even if a restaurant advertises "no trans fat," you still need to be cautious in your food selection. Restaurants replace trans fats with other types of fats and oils, which have roughly the same number of calories as trans fats. When eating out, look at all nutritional information provided for foods, including the total number of calories, fat calories, sodium, and refined sugars.

Polyunsaturated fats: Polyunsaturated fats come from vegetable oils such as safflower, corn, sunflower, soy, and cottonseed. Nuts and seeds are also a source of polyunsaturated fats. Pay particular attention to omega-3 fatty acids, a type of polyunsaturated fat. The AHA indicates that this fat appears to lessen the risk of artery disease and to help lower blood pressure. Omega-3 fatty acids are found primarily in cold-water fish such as salmon, mackerel, and herring. Flaxseeds, flaxseed oil, and walnuts are also good sources of omega-3 fatty acids. Omega-6 fatty acids are present in nuts, seeds, and the oils that we derive from nuts.

Other Label Ingredients

While you can certainly lose weight by controlling your calorie intake, you might be doing yourself a disservice if you fail to take into account the overall nutritional value of the foods you eat. Nutritional labels give you a wealth of information, assuming you know what to look for.

Fiber

Fiber aids in digestion and lowers the risk of diabetes and heart disease. A high-fiber food contains 5 grams of fiber or more per serving. The 2010 USDA *Dietary Guidelines for Americans* recommends that men age fifty and under eat at least 38 grams of fiber per day, while women age fifty and under should consume at least 25 grams of fiber per day. If a man is over fifty, he needs 28 grams of fiber; a woman over fifty requires 22 grams. Fresh and dried fruits contain fiber, while canned fruits are generally devoid of fiber. Other sources of fiber include vegetables and whole grains such as popcorn, oatmeal, whole wheat, quinoa, brown rice, millet, rye, and buckwheat. Look for the words "whole grain" or "whole wheat" on package labels.

Vitamins and Minerals

At a minimum, the standard nutrition label lists vitamin A, vitamin C, calcium, and iron. To find the complete nutritional information for foods, use a reputable Web site, such as the USDA's Nutrient Data Laboratory site, which allows you to search for thousands of foods. Eating a well-balanced diet that gives you all the vitamins and minerals you need is relatively easy when you eat a variety of foods from the five food groups (grains, vegetables, fruits, protein, and dairy) and avoid a diet high in processed foods.

Sodium

High amounts of sodium (salt) in your diet can increase your risk of high blood pressure. Try to limit your sodium intake to 1,500 milligrams (mg) per day. This can be very difficult if you regularly eat processed foods. Cereals, crackers, canned soups and beans, and baked chips all contain high amounts of sodium. If you eat a lot of processed food, you will quickly exceed the recommended sodium intake for the day. For example, five snack crackers have 141 mg of sodium, which is 9.4 percent of your daily requirement, and 1 cup of low-calorie garden vegetable soup has 480 mg, which is 32 percent of your daily requirement. Restaurant foods can have unhealthy levels of sodium even if the calories and fat percentages are low. For example, a 6-inch turkey submarine sandwich from a popular fast-food restaurant has more than 800 mg of sodium.

Low Fat Does Not Always Save Calories

In a majority of foods, the calorie difference between the low-fat and the regular version is minor. The following list shows the fat percentages and calorie counts of some popular low-fat and regular food items.

Food	Calories per Serving	Fat Percentage
Reduced-fat crackers	70	30
Regular crackers	80	50
Low-fat graham crackers	120	12
Regular graham crackers	130	23
Light ranch dressing	80	88
Regular ranch dressing	140	93
Reduced-fat cream of mushroom soup	70	29
Regular cream of mushroom soup	100	54
Reduced-fat biscuit mix	140	16
Regular biscuit mix	160	34

A bit surprising, isn't it? When food manufacturers reformulate their products to lower-fat versions, they often replace fat with sugar. Sugar contains no fat and 4 calories per gram, as opposed to 9 calories per gram for fat. So the calorie difference between low-fat crackers and regular crackers, for instance, is small—only 10 calories. When I was obese and would eat entire sleeves of crackers at one time, I would justify it by reasoning that they were low fat and okay to eat. I was right—they were okay to eat. It just wasn't okay to eat half the box.

Now that you are a math whiz and a label-reading pro, it's time to focus on portion size, the second facet of Fit to the Finish.

6

Portion Importance

Portion control is of vital importance to the Fit to the Finish weight-loss plan. Even if you religiously watch your overall fat intake and exercise regularly, you will have difficulty losing weight if you fail to control portion size.

I was a portion girl—a big-portion girl. Why buy the king-size candy bar when for a few cents more I could get the mammoth, family-size bar? At dinner at home, I'd give myself the biggest portion of the most fattening foods. Who got the extra fries? Me. The winner of the biggest bowl of ice cream? Me. In teaching my classes and talking with people, I've come to realize I'm not alone. Portion control is hard. In our supersize world, big food is in. It's difficult to go against the tide and eat the proper amount of food, whether you are at home or in a restaurant. But you can make the change. It just takes some practice.

From a theoretical point of view, I find the portion sizes of packaged foods to be very interesting. I invite you to go to your pantry right now and check out the calorie count on the sides of the boxes and cans. You will find the majority of foods you buy have roughly 120 to 220 calories per serving, even though the food items are vastly different.

A few hundred calories. Goodness, that isn't much, is it? A low calorie count on the label appeals to consumers, so food manufacturers oblige us by adjusting serving sizes down—so the calories per serving are reasonable. If the calories listed on the box are low, we assume the food is not going to fatten us up.

A good example of serving size distortion is cereal. Some cereal boxes in my pantry list serving sizes of 1/2 cup. Others list serving sizes of 3/4 cup or 1 cup. Even a 1-cup serving appears awfully small when poured into a bowl. When I was losing weight, I measured out a serving of cereal and was shocked at how small it was. I realized I had been consuming three or four servings of dry cereal for a morning snack. No wonder I was gaining weight!

Quantity Was Important to Me

When I was fat, I paid little attention to the serving sizes on nutrition labels. Honestly, I rarely looked at labels at all. Even when I was supposed to be dieting, nutrition-label reading was low on my list of priorities. Why read the label when you can just look at the picture? I had reached the point where the quantity of the food I was eating was more important than the quality.

I selected restaurant meals based on the size of the entrée, and I did the same with packaged foods. If a cracker box came with four sleeves of crackers, I figured each sleeve was probably a serving. If I ate two sleeves, that was two servings, right?

I tried to justify my huge portions by rationalizing: *Well, there are just 70 calories per serving in these crackers, so that's not too bad for me.* I never looked at the serving size but focused only on the calories. If I had taken a minute, I would have seen that the serving size was five crackers, not fifty. Instead of eating just 70 calories, I easily consumed 700 calories in less than thirty minutes. Those 700 calories were more than a third of my total daily requirement.

I couldn't control myself around potato chips. Forget the little single serving bags sold at the convenience store. I wanted the big bag, and I didn't want to share either. Many times I'd stick the whole chip bag in my purse and repeatedly put my hand in there for some nourishment while I was driving down the road. The challenge was to only use one hand, so I wouldn't spread grease all over the steering wheel.

I was sad to discover that a typical serving of chips is about 1 ounce, or thirteen to fifteen chips. Not enough for me. But I adjusted to the lower amount and bought baked chips instead. One day, just for fun, I put an

---

One Serving at a Time?

Watching portions is easy in theory, but when you are staring at a plateful of cookies or looking at your favorite pie sitting on the counter, controlling portion size suddenly becomes much more difficult. It's easy to look at a label and see the recommended portion size, but it can be hard to eat just one serving.

Before I finally got serious about losing weight, I cheated on portion sizes all the time. I'd count out one serving of crackers. After I had eaten that, I'd take out another serving. Once when I had counted out animal cookies for the fourth time, John came in and said, "Good for you for counting out how many you should have." I nodded, my mouth full of the fiftieth and fifty-first cookies. After he left the room, I calmly finished my fourth portion and counted out fourteen more cookies. This didn't do a whole lot for my weight-loss efforts.

The key to portion control is training yourself to be satisfied with just one serving at a time. If you are having a sandwich, crackers, fruit, carrots, and yogurt for lunch, then that is all you can have. You can't go back to the cracker box time and time again and expect to lose weight. Believe me, I know. I tried it.

---

open bag of chips on the counter and invited the kids to have some. They reached their hands in, and each pulled out a good-size handful. My four-year-old ended up with ten chips, and my twelve-year-old old scored sixteen. Unlike me, the girls were very happy with the chips they grabbed and did not ask for more after they ate their treat. How many handfuls of chips do you usually eat at one time? I could never eat just one handful. If I tried to limit the amount I ate, I felt unsatisfied.

Although serving sizes are often small, you can use that to your advantage in controlling your calories. You may not normally eat just five crackers, two cookies, or 1 tablespoon of dressing, but you can follow the recommended serving sizes to reduce your caloric intake throughout the day. Do a better job of controlling your portions and you take a giant leap in the right direction.

Portion control trips up more people than fat percentage. The participants in my classes quickly adjust their food choices to lower-fat options but often aren't satisfied after eating just one portion of food. It was hard for me to go from eating as much as I could possibly stuff in my mouth to eating just one portion too. I just kept telling myself, *One is all you need, and one is all you get.*

How Much Is Too Much?

A funny thing happened to John and me recently. It was the anniversary of our engagement, and we decided to go to Olive Garden for lunch. After looking over the menu, John decided to order one of the healthy entrées. When his food came, he looked at me and said, "That's not a very big piece of chicken is it?" I said, "No, but that's actually the right size piece of meat." Being accustomed to gigantic restaurant portions, he was not too impressed by the size of that chicken, but he ate it anyway. When he finished his meal, he remarked that he was pleasantly full, not overstuffed like he usually was after eating at a restaurant.

As an obese person, I was accustomed to eating large quantities of high-fat food. When I first started trying to lose weight and get fit, I didn't know what the standard serving sizes of certain foods actually were. I made a concerted effort to measure foods, to look at pictures of portion sizes in books, and to use a USDA Web page that shows the standard serving sizes for many foods. According to the USDA, here are the proper portion sizes for some common foods:

Whole-grain bread: 1 slice
Diet bread: 2 slices
Cooked rice or pasta: 1/2 c
Mashed potatoes: 1/2 c
Baked potato: 1 (small)
Crackers: 3–4 (small)
Cookies: 2 (medium size)
Pancakes or waffles: 2 (small)
Cooked vegetables: 1/2 c
Lettuce: 4 leaves

Vegetable juice: 3/4 c
Apple: 1 (medium)
Grapefruit: 1/2
Berries: 1 c
Yogurt or milk: 1 c
Cheese: 1 1/2 oz
Chicken breast: 1 (3 oz)
Pork chop: 1 (medium)
Hamburger patty: 1/4 lb (4 oz)

Practice, Practice, Practice

Instead of remembering all the numbers associated with each portion, I find it easier to visualize each portion. The next time you make rice or pasta, use a measuring cup to spoon 1/2 cup onto your plate. After you get over the shock at how small it looks, remember that amount for next time.

When working on portion control, spend a week or two making friends with your measuring cups and spoons. If you take time to measure the proper portions, you will be an expert in no time. You can also use visual clues to remember portion sizes. Here are some common visual cues:

- A serving of vegetables or fruits is the size of your fist.
- A serving of cooked pasta or rice is as big as a scoop of ice cream.
- Beef, fish, and chicken pieces are about the size of the palm of your hand.
- Servings of pretzels, chips, and snack crackers are about the size of a cupped handful (don't cheat).
- A proper-size baked sweet or white potato is the size of a computer mouse.
- Bagels should be the size of a hockey puck—not a Frisbee.
- A portion of cheese is about as long as your thumb, or two dice put together.

Mastering Portion Control

Before, if you had asked me if it were possible to eat Dove chocolate in moderation, I would have laughed my head off. I thought moderation was impossible for me, but I learned I could moderate what I ate. With practice, I quickly became an expert at recognizing proper-size portions. And I was pleasantly surprised when I realized that portion control actually gave me the freedom to eat a wider variety of foods. Instead of stuffing my face with hordes of chips and not much else in a fruitless attempt to control my calories, I could have fruits, breads, a few baked chips, a healthy dinner, and even a small snack. Who knew? Instead of limiting my choices, portion control increased them.

I spent a lot of days as an overweight and obese person feeling guilty because of my poor eating habits. By making portion control part of my daily routine, I was able to put the feelings of guilt aside. Now I don't feel guilty eating a small piece of candy because I know it fits within my daily fat and calorie allotment.

Once you master portion sizes, you will feel a freedom you may have never known. An increased feeling of freedom came over me on Thanksgiving during my weight-loss year. I ate a piece of pie, with whipped cream, without feeling guilty. I may have still wanted the whole pie, but one piece satisfied me. Before, I would have continually gone back to the pie, cutting off tiny sliver after tiny sliver until the pie was gone. And every time I stuffed a tiny piece in my mouth, I would feel guilty. But that Thanksgiving, for the first time in a decade, I had no guilt over my choice. Portion control isn't something to fear but something to embrace.

So often we associate limiting our portions with deprivation. Nothing could be further from the truth. Over time, I hope you feel as I do and realize that portion control gives you freedom from guilt and opens the door to experimenting with new healthier foods.

In developing Fit to the Finish, I realized that portion size and fat percentage go hand in hand. If the fat percentage of the food you want to eat is acceptable, and you just eat one portion, then your calories and fat grams will fall in line all by themselves, especially if you include lots of vegetables in your daily diet.

Too Simple?

If you think watching portions and fat percentage is almost too simple, you're right. I developed Fit to the Finish because I wanted something easy enough to follow my whole life, without constantly having to look up calories or count fat grams. While you may need to initially familiarize yourself with portion sizes, calorie amounts, and foods with too much unhealthy fat, over time these techniques will become second nature to you. After thirteen years of weight maintenance, I need to spend very little time researching foods. I know it seems simple, but eating proper portion sizes, coupled with appropriate fat percentages, will reduce your calories to a level that is appropriate for weight loss.

7

Let's Get Moving

Exercise is not a four-letter word, although if you had asked me about it fourteen years ago, I may have told you it was. My idea of exercise was hauling myself off the couch and walking to the pantry and back. All the better if I could get one of the children or John to just bring me food. God forbid if I had to pick myself up off the couch and answer the phone. Television remotes, cordless phones, and TV trays were very good friends of mine. I never expended any unnecessary energy.

Fit to the Finish works best if you take advantage of all three components, including exercise. While losing weight can occur by simply creating a deficit between how many calories your body requires to function and how many calories you consume, not including exercise in your weight-loss plan robs you of several crucial benefits. As I lost weight using my plan, I realized that when I exercised, I was less likely to eat a cookie or an unhealthy snack because I did not want to eat back the calories I had burned. I also revved up my metabolism each day by exercising regularly, and I enjoyed the mental satisfaction of accomplishing physical tasks that had previously seemed beyond my reach.

I hadn't always been lazy. But the more weight I carried, the less active I became. I hadn't yet become housebound, but I was probably on my way. And while I was busy sitting my life away, I always had food to keep me company.

As much as I loved food, I hated exercise. No matter how much free time I had or how much weight I gained, it never crossed my mind to get off the couch and move. After all, who had time to exercise? I had time to watch television, surf the Internet, talk on the phone, and eat, but no time to carve out thirty minutes a day for exercise. Besides, I was sure exercise wouldn't make a difference in my weight anyway. Oh, was I wrong. Once I actually started exercising, instead of just making fun of people who did, I was amazed at how I felt. I felt empowered.

My first exercise was walking. At the time, I weighed almost 300 pounds, and putting one foot in front of the other with neither refrigerator nor television in sight wasn't easy. At first I felt I might pass out with every other step. To my surprise, within just six weeks, I was walking 2 miles up and down the hills of our neighborhood. By the end of the first year, I could jog 3 miles. It was a major victory the first time I ran a 5k race. I'll never forget John, Rachel, Grace, and baby Mark smiling at me when I crossed the finish line. What a great memory. I'm so glad that I quit making excuses and gave it a try.

We have all read the books, magazines, and newspaper articles extolling the virtues of exercise. We know it improves our health, enhances our mood, and helps us lose and maintain weight. And believe it or not, exercise can be fun. Why, then, can't the majority of us seem to incorporate a consistent time for exercise into our day? Why do so many of us think of exercise as an activity best avoided?

There are thousands of excuses for not exercising, but there is only one reason not to. If your doctor says don't, then don't. But do ask your doctor whether you can do gentle exercise such as yoga or water aerobics.

Your Turn

What stops you from exercising? Check all that apply:

❏ Work	❏ Money	❏ Health
❏ Kids	❏ Lack of energy	❏ Worries
❏ Spouse	❏ Fear	❏ Time
❏ Significant other	❏ Feelings	

Have you ever exercised in the past? ....Yes ❏ No ❏

How long ago? _____

_____

What type of exercise did you do? _____

_____

_____

How often did you exercise? _____

_____

_____

How did it make you feel? _____

_____

_____

Did you enjoy athletics when you were younger? .... Yes ❑ No ❑

If yes, what type of activities did you enjoy? _____

_____

_____

These questions can be difficult. When I answered them, I could remember enjoying some activities but couldn't imagine participating in them as an obese woman. It made me sad to think about times I had passed up school field trips with my daughter because I wasn't physically capable. If you regret missing out on things because of your weight, work to put those feelings aside. Instead, focus on the amazing results you can achieve by committing to an exercise program.

Day-to-Day Living Was Hard

Before I started the Fit to the Finish plan, my fitness level was dismal. Even simple activities were hard. It was physically difficult to climb stairs. I avoided them whenever I could.

One day, while visiting a friend in Atlanta, I agreed to head to the mall with her for some retail therapy. At the time, I weighed well above 250 pounds. I was beginning to experience joint pain when I walked. On this particular day, I was determined to keep up with my average-size friend and not to sit down to rest as I usually did when I shopped with my family.

We wandered in and out of stores, examining clothes that would fit her but that I couldn't get my right calf in. Before long, I thought I was going to die. My legs hurt, I was tired, my feet hurt, and I was done. Finally, she said the magic words: "Hey, there's a great little coffee shop here. Do you want to get some coffee?"

If I could have, I would have jumped up and down with excitement, but I just calmly said, "That sounds good." She and I began walking, and walking, and walking. Along the way, we passed comfortable chairs and benches, all calling my name. "Sit down, Diane. Sit down." But I didn't. I just kept walking. She finally pointed up and said, "There it is."

I looked up, and looming ahead was the longest flight of stairs I had seen in a long time. They seemed to extend forever. If I used bad language, this would again be where I'd put it. *You've got to be kidding,* I thought. *There is no way I can do those stairs after walking around for over an hour.* But I just smiled and followed her. She walked up the stairs like a normal person, barely touching the rail, and I started up after her. Step by step, I moved up, sliding my hand up the rail before my body, trying to get some leverage.

She turned around and said, "You okay?" I nodded, not able to speak. I finally got up the stairs, and to my embarrassment, and partial relief, she said, "Why don't we sit here. I'll check in at home." She could see I was out of breath. I probably looked like I was in pain. We sat on the bench for a few minutes while she made her unnecessary phone call.

While sitting on the bench, I tried to surreptitiously catch my breath but finally found myself inhaling and exhaling loudly to breathe easier. There, I had done it. I could talk again. I was embarrassed and frustrated. I jokingly told my friend, "Next time, I'll find the elevator, and I'll meet you up here!" We both laughed at my funny joke, but inside I was mortified. *How in the world could this have happened to me?* We eventually got off the bench and walked over to the coffee shop, where I ordered only coffee. If I hadn't just embarrassed myself by barely being able to walk up the stairs, I would have ordered a sticky bun as well.

We enjoyed our time at the mall, and although she may not remember that particular event, it is branded in my mind. I was twenty-nine, fat, and unhappy. I had gone from average size to obese, reasonably fit to out of shape, and had seen my self-confidence plummet. It would be two more years before I finally was able to start losing weight and get fit. Those next two years were filled with more embarrassing situations like the one at the mall.

Your Turn

Where are you today in terms of avoiding physical activity? _____
_____
_____
_____

Do you avoid the stairs in front of you and opt to find the hidden elevator?
_____
_____
_____

Stuck at Disney World

During my ten years of obesity, I avoided expending any unnecessary energy, but we still functioned as a regular family. We threw the kids birthday parties, attended church socials, went on trips to the park, and occasionally visited the beach. We even managed to take two trips to Disney World.

It was 1996. Rachel was six and Grace was three. We loaded up the van early one morning and drove to Orlando. The anticipation of seeing Mickey Mouse was almost more than the four of us could bear. After a few bathroom breaks, we arrived at Disney World and parked the car in the vast lot. Once inside the park, John and I both loved seeing the girls' reaction to the magic of Disney World.

At the time I weighed more than 280 pounds and wore a size 26/28. I wore a pair of home-sewn white cotton capri pants and a pink-and-white-striped "big shirt"—so large that it dropped from the shoulders with no defined shape. It was kind of like a big paper bag, except with sleeves. I suppose I looked as nice as I could for my size, but I didn't feel good about myself that morning.

So there we were at Disney World with our daughters. It was a magical time for the first two hours, but by 11:00 a.m., I was completely exhausted. I remember standing in Fantasyland, looking at the long line for Dumbo the Flying Elephant. There was no way I could physically stand in one more line. I looked at John and told him to go on the ride without me. He said, "You're not going to come on Dumbo?" I said, "No, I don't think I can. I just need to rest a few minutes." He offered to wait, but I persuaded him to go. He reluctantly stood in line and rode with the girls. I can't tell you how bad I felt watching them fly through the air without me. I was in denial that any of the fatigue I felt was due to my obesity. I just thought perhaps I didn't have as much energy as other people.

Disney World was more than just a tiring physical experience for me; it was also a humiliating experience. I refused to go on some rides because I was afraid I wouldn't fit. I didn't know if the park had accommodations for overweight people, and I wasn't about to ask! When it was time to ride Peter Pan, I told John it was too scary for the girls. It may have been, but I was really afraid I wouldn't fit behind the bar that automatically comes down over your hips, and I was probably right.

I did summon up the courage to attempt the carousel. When it was our turn to ride, I selected a beautiful white horse with a flowing plastic mane and hauled myself up onto its back. Hauling more than 250 pounds several feet in the air was a major accomplishment for someone so out of shape, but it was worth the effort. It was the one ride I didn't want to come down from. Rachel, Grace, and John loved the merry-go-round too, and I loved

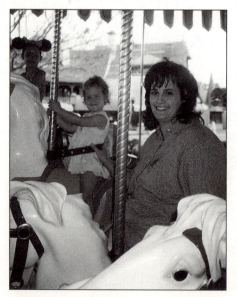

being with them. The problem came when the ride stopped. My beautiful horse, which had been so obliging when I boarded, had stubbornly ended in an up position, and no matter how much I wished for him to come down, he stayed right where he was. I grabbed that brass pole with all my strength and put my weight on my left foot. I tried to slide

I enjoyed feeling like I was almost weightless as I rode the carousel horse. I panicked when I realized I had to get off.

my right foot out of the stirrup, but it wouldn't budge. The lower half of my body was so heavy that I could not move. I tried again. I took my right foot out first and tried to balance on my left foot. That worked until I realized that I couldn't swing my right foot high enough to clear the horse's behind. I was stuck.

At this point, John noticed I was still sitting on the white horse, suspended in the air like a marionette. It wasn't good. He came over, bringing the girls with him, and said, "What's the matter? Can't you get down?" I shook my head no. Somehow, with his help I managed to slide off the horse. That was one situation I will never forget and never want to experience again. The rest of the day passed by in a blur. All I could think about was getting stuck on the carousel. *Why do things like this have to happen to me? What have I done to deserve this?* Never once did I take responsibility for my physical predicaments.

As we left the park, I looked back at Cinderella Castle, knowing that just beyond it lay the carousel and the memory of one more embarrassing moment. But as an encouragement to you, here's a picture of me a few years later on the same carousel, but 150 pounds lighter.

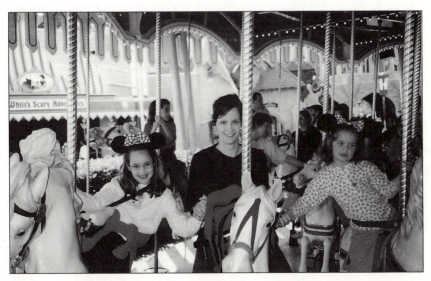

The contrast between the two visits to Disney World is summed up in this picture. Here I was confident, carefree, and not worried about whether I could get off my horse.

Your Turn

Are you able to accept responsibility for your physical
limitations? .... Yes ❑ No ❑

What role does denial play in your ability to perpetuate your inactivity
and to avoid taking responsibility for your physical fitness level? _____

_____

_____

_____

_____

Why Exercise?

Even though I had a tendency to blame fate for the embarrassing weight-
related incidents in my life, I knew I should be moving my body. I knew
I should be eating better. I knew weighing so much wasn't good for me.
Why didn't I just exercise? Why couldn't I control this part of my life? I
knew the benefits exercise offered, understood I was obese, yet couldn't
seem to get off the couch. The thought of putting on a pair of shorts and
lumbering into a gym or walking down my own road struck terror in my
heart. Rather than face the possibility of feeling uncomfortable, I sat.

According to studies, regular exercise offers many benefits. They
include the following:

- Reduced risk of premature death
- Reduced risk of developing and dying from heart disease
- Reduced blood pressure and risk of developing high blood pressure
- Reduced cholesterol and risk of developing high cholesterol
- Reduced risk of developing colon and breast cancer
- Reduced risk of developing diabetes
- Reduced body weight and body fat
- Healthier muscles, bones, and joints
- Reduced depression and anxiety
- Improved psychological well-being
- Enhanced work, recreation, and sports performance

If exercise is so beneficial, why do only about 30 percent of Americans exercise for at least thirty minutes a day, five days a week? If you are one of the approximately 70 percent of Americans who choose not to exercise regularly, Why not?

Barbara was in my Fit to the Finish weight-loss class several years ago. She, like many of you, had slowly gained weight over the years, until she was approximately 75 pounds overweight. She had stopped chaperoning her children's field trips because of her embarrassment over her weight. She made excuses, and instead of spending that time with her children, she stayed home and made cookies. She felt paralyzed by worry anytime she had to exert herself physically. What if she could not keep up with everyone else? What if she further embarrassed her children? I encouraged her to start walking as part of the plan, and after a few weeks she did. She later shared with the class her initial fears and how she felt the first time she took a walk for exercise. *Tired* and *sweaty* were two of the words she used, but she also included the words *proud* and *motivated*. Exercise wasn't so bad after all, even with a significant amount of weight to lose.

Your Turn

List every emotional benefit you can think of that might occur when you exercise (for example, ability to handle stress, improved mood). _____
_____

When your emotional health is strong, how do you feel? _____
_____
_____

How does your emotional well-being influence your actions? _____
_____
_____

How does your household function when you are feeling good about yourself emotionally? _____
_____

If exercise can help regulate your emotions, why do you not take the time to exercise on a regular basis? _____

_____

_____

Will you commit to some form of exercise? .... Yes ❑ No ❑

Can you easily (check all that apply):
❑ Run a short distance?   ❑ Be on your feet for long periods?
❑ Walk for an hour at a time?   ❑ Keep up with children on a hike?
❑ Climb several flights of stairs?

Who, Me?

At no point during the years I was fat did I ever consider that a small change in lifestyle would make a difference. I felt the change had to be all or nothing. Looking back, if I had attempted only to improve my fitness level, I would have begun to feel better about myself. As it was, I was tired physically, depressed, and struggling with self-esteem. I let my weight get out of control by making choices (on a daily basis) that were detrimental to my body. I paid the price for those choices physically and emotionally. I allowed myself to become dangerously obese.

Do you know the definition of obesity? The clinical definition of obesity is a body mass index (BMI) of 30 or higher, which translates to being 20 percent over your ideal body weight. Morbid obesity occurs when you are 100 percent over your ideal body weight. Because I weighed twice what I should have, I was morbidly obese. A person who is morbidly obese has a greater risk of respiratory problems, cardiovascular disease, unhealthy cholesterol levels, high blood pressure, and an increased risk of death.

If you aren't sure whether your current weight places you in the category of normal, overweight, obese, or morbidly obese, see the BMI chart in appendix D. Find your height on the top of chart and your weight on the left side of chart. Then slide your fingers down and across until you reach the intersection of your height and weight. The number where the two lines meet is your BMI. Also refer to these BMI classifications:

Underweight: BMI less than 19
Normal: BMI between 19 and 24.9
Overweight: BMI between 25 and 29.9
Obese: BMI between 30 and 34.9
Severely obese: BMI between 35 and 39.9
Morbidly Obese: BMI between 40 and 49.9
Super obese: BMI greater than 50

Obese is not a pretty word—not to say, not to write, and definitely not to see applied to you. The first time someone applied the word *obese* to me was at a doctor's appointment for one of my pregnancies. The nurse was prattling on about something, and I was busy reading my chart upside down. I saw all the vital statistics and then a row of boxes with various check marks. Curious, I examined which boxes the nurse had checked. There it was in black and white—a check mark by that vile word: obese. I could not believe it. I knew I was heavy. Okay, fat. But obese? Obese was for people who had to ride in carts in the grocery store, not for a young twentysomething mom to be!

The nurse and my doctor knew what I could not admit. I was medically obese. The rest of the appointment passed in a blur. The doctor talked on and on, and I responded automatically, all the while my mind reeling. *What exactly did obese mean? Why did it matter?*

As soon as I got home, I fired up the Internet, did some research, and found that, yes, I was not only obese but morbidly obese. With a height of 70 inches and a high weight of 305, my BMI was 44.4. With that number, I was morbidly obese. Sounds really great, doesn't it?

I discovered that for my height, my maximum weight should have been 174. Even being generous with the maximum weight, 20 percent over 174 was 209. I was so far above the "obese" level of 209 that I couldn't even fathom how to go about losing well over 100 pounds.

I wish I could say that learning I was officially obese sent me running down the road in an exercise frenzy, but the revelation sent me running to the grocery store for cookies and chocolate. I was depressed about my physical health and could not figure out how to improve it, or to find the motivation to change. I sat on the couch and contemplated that problem. Somewhere in my heart, the desire to get healthier was there, but it wasn't yet strong enough to move me in the right direction.

Your Turn

Where are you? Use the BMI classifications above and the BMI chart in appendix D to determine your status.

You current weight: _____

Your normal BMI weight range: _____

Your BMI: _____

Your BMI classification: _____

Are you obese?.. Yes ❑ No ❑

If you are obese, how does that make you feel? _____
_____
_____
_____

Perhaps you are realizing for the first time that you are medically obese. Or maybe you have just a few pounds to lose. Either way, just acknowledging where you are right now is a wonderful first step.

Stepping Out

In 1997, when I finally got serious about my weight loss, what did I do for exercise? How did I go from being stuck on the carousel at Disney World to being able to complete a 5k at a slow but steady jog? After deciding what foods to eat (*see* chapters 4, 5, and 6) based on fat percentage and committing to eating one portion at a time, I knew (from the many books I had read and from finally listening to my doctor's advice) that I needed to add exercise to my personal plan. I committed myself to daily exercise. I did not write down my exercise commitment as I had my healthy eating commitment. I just purposed in my heart that exercise was going to be part of my new lifestyle.

I chose to exercise every day for accountability. It was too easy to say, "Well, I'm going to exercise three times this week. I will exercise on Mondays, Wednesdays, and Fridays and take the other four days off." Eons before, when I had tried the three-day-a-week approach, I discovered it didn't work for me. I might exercise on Monday but then on Wednesday something would come up, so I wouldn't exercise. Then by Friday I was too tired, and I reasoned that since I had exercised only once that week, I might as well wait until the following Monday to begin again. Then the next Monday would roll around, and I would remember all the bad food I had eaten over the weekend, so I didn't exercise Monday either. Does this scenario sound familiar to you? I cannot tell you how many times I would begin a diet, think about exercising, and never follow through. I also thought, "Well it's so hard to cut back on eating. Trying to start an exercise program at the same time is too much at once."

When I began my lifestyle change the final time, I committed to daily exercise and drastically altered my food consumption. I had self-discipline in many areas of life, but I had never been disciplined when it came to eating and exercise. If I could apply discipline and self-control to my work life, my housework, and my social life, why had I never been able to conquer my weight? This time was different because I approached weight loss and exercise like I did my work. Follow-through and commitment were of paramount importance. Therefore, I did not allow myself much leeway when it came to exercise. The days I missed my exercise program were few and far between.

Your Turn

Can you make a commitment to regular exercise?................ Yes ❑ No ❑

Will you put your commitment in writing? .... Yes ❑ No ❑

Will you treat your commitment to yourself like a
work contract?... Yes ❑ No ❑

What days of the week will you commit to exercising? _____
_____

What other commitments do you already succeed in keeping? Think about your parenting responsibilities, work-related activities, charitable activities, and hobbies. _____

_____

_____

_____

Don't Let Anything Stand in Your Way

Here's a picture of me in 1994—the last time I wore shorts during my obesity. It was hard to be shortless in the Florida summer, but I did it for several years. By 1997 I wore dresses or jumpers year-round and on occasion my one pair of big-girl jeans. Sometimes people asked if I was hot in my jeans. I would lie and say, "Oh, no. I like to wear pants." I would continue the thought silently in my mind, saying, *Oh, no. I like to wear pants in 100-degree weather, feeling the sweat drip down my legs into my shoes.*

When I began walking in the spring of 1997, I wore jumpers. I had jumpers in every style and fabric. All were equally unattractive, but for the first time in my adult life, I was motivated to move, and I was not going

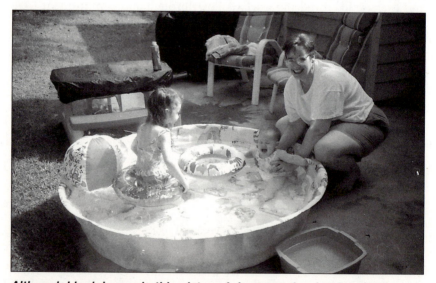

Although I look happy in this picture, I do remember hoping that I wouldn't fall over when I tried to get up from this squatting position.

to let clothing or anything else stand in my way. I could have let a lack of appropriate exercise attire become an obstacle. But I didn't. I worked with or around this and other obstacles, including out-of-town company, family obligations, and illness.

In spite of all the obstacles in life, it is always possible to carve out some time to exercise. You might have to ask your family for help in scheduling time. Making time might require some sacrifice on your part, or on the part of others. As you think about when to fit in a time for exercise, keep in mind that all of us waste time, usually watching television or surfing the Internet.

I needed at least thirty minutes a day for exercise, and I had to decide what activity to borrow the time from. I borrowed the time from sleep. I decided to exercise first thing in the morning, before John left for work. Because I had young children who could not be left alone while I took a walk, I needed to finish my exercise while John was home. That meant I needed to be out the door by 6:15 a.m. I had to get up at 6:00, much earlier than normal. Exercising first thing in the morning also meant I didn't have the entire day to talk myself out of it. Getting up earlier wasn't easy, but it wasn't impossible either.

I didn't exercise vigorously at first. I walked ten minutes away from my house and ten minutes back each morning, but I couldn't believe how different I felt. My minimal effort brought a big payoff, including increased energy, firmer muscles, looser clothing, and a sense of accomplishment.

Your Turn

Think about your average day. How many different roles do you play (for example, chauffeur, cook, executive, vet, doctor)? _____

_____

_____

_____

What obstacles might prevent you from starting, maintaining, or increasing the intensity of an exercise program? _____

_____

_____

_____

What obstacles can you remove, ignore, or overcome this week? _____
_____
_____

What will you do when you confront your obstacles? _____
_____
_____

Can you ask a family member to help you?............................ Yes ❑ No ❑

Do you have a friend who might want to begin an exercise program with you? _____
_____

What activities could you borrow some time from during the day? _____
_____
_____

Do you need to change your schedule to fit in time to
exercise? .... Yes ❑ No ❑

Can you do this?.. Yes ❑ No ❑

In the Land of the Fit

The first morning of my new life, I woke up early and put on my home-made jumper. Once outside, my old white tennis shoes padded silently on the neighborhood road. In the quiet of the morning, I could hear my breath huffing and puffing as I plodded down my street. I'm sure I was quite a sight to see, but I didn't care. The first day I walked, I was extremely proud of myself. When I got home twenty minutes later and collapsed on the couch, I told my husband I was now among those in the "land of the fit." Every time I talked with him on the phone that day, I asked if he was proud of me for getting up early and walking. Each time he would say, "Yes, yes, yes." I'm sure he was tired of hearing me brag about my one day of exercise, but he was encouraging.

For me, a morbidly obese woman, walking for exercise was hard. I came home hot, sweaty, and out of breath. But I also came home with an incredible sense of accomplishment and the feeling that I was finally on my way to looking better and feeling good about myself. I made it a point to remember that feeling. Before long, the thought of not having time to do my walk was worse than the thought of doing it.

Your Turn

If you have not exercised recently, how do you think you will feel when you start? _____

_____

_____

How has exercise made you feel in the past? _____

_____

_____

Who will you share your victory story with? _____

_____

Fitness Came Quickly

For many years I hated how I looked. I gave up on trying to look cute and fabulous. After all, who looks at the fat girl in the room? I felt like no matter what I did to look better, I would still be fat. My new exercise program gave me such a good feeling that I started to pay attention to how I looked, to wear a little bit of makeup, and to think about the day when I would be able to buy clothes in a department store again.

After just three weeks, I could walk for thirty minutes each day, including hills. Our neighborhood back then was quite hilly, and our house was on the top of three hills that converged at our driveway. So no matter which way I went, I had to come uphill at the end of my walk. At first, that was a challenge of monumental proportions. I would huff and puff my way up the hill, leaning forward as I went, thinking, *I have to do this.*

I would count the number of houses until I reached ours. Once I hit the white house down the road, I knew I was only eight houses away. Every time I got up the hill, I felt a sense of pride.

In a previous question set, I asked you to list some obstacles that have kept you from beginning or restarting an exercise program. I could have let the three children be an excuse, but I didn't. Although I preferred to walk in the morning, before John left for work, sometimes that wasn't convenient for his schedule. On days when he had to leave for work early or go out of town, I still exercised.

The first day it happened, I panicked a little. How would I get my walk in with three small children? I did not normally take the children with me when I walked for exercise. Honestly, I enjoyed the time alone, when I could think about my day, focus on how fast I was walking, and have some "me time." However, that morning I was determined not to let a scheduling conflict derail my plans. After breakfast, I put the two little ones in my largest single stroller and got Rachel ready to ride her bike. Rachel was excited to be going on a bike ride in the morning. She bounced up and down on her little bicycle seat. Grace was happy as usual, and Mark was satisfied with his "baba." Before we went down the road, I explained to Rachel that she would need to stop at each intersection so that we could turn or cross together. She felt like such a big girl. It was a great experience for the four of us.

No Going Back, No More Excuses

Realizing I was still exercising in my jumpers, a friend gave me an early birthday present: a Just My Size 3X shorts/shirt set. I was grateful not have to wear my jumpers any longer and wore those teal green shorts every day. (I washed them frequently.) I didn't let the clothes be an obstacle. I didn't let the children be an obstacle. I didn't let the time factor be an obstacle. I also didn't let my moods be an obstacle. If it was a hormonally challenging time of the month for me, I went anyway. If I had a head cold, I went anyway. If it was cold or rainy, I went anyway. Did I ever regret exercising? Never. I subscribed to the five-minute rule. If you aren't sure you want to exercise, go for five minutes. If at the end of five minutes you feel worse, then stop. If I was a little under the weather, I would go slowly, always mindful of exercising within my fitness and health level.

Once I started exercising, I was able to stay on my feet, running after the kids throughout the day without sitting down, make a healthy dinner, and spend time with John in the evening without falling asleep. At first I worried that exercise would make me tired and burned out, but the opposite happened. Exercise energized me, and I started to enjoy exercising. I liked the way it made me feel physically and emotionally. My outlook on life improved dramatically. I became more positive and looked at life from a healthier perspective. I no longer filtered every opportunity to be physically active through the "I can't do it because I'm fat" mentality. I gradually increased the time I spent exercising until I was walking between thirty and forty-five minutes each day. Instead of dreading the hills, I started looking forward to the challenge they offered. My breathing became less labored. I stopped getting winded when I had to climb stairs.

And I saw my body change in dramatic ways. It changed much more quickly than it had when I had dieted but not exercised. Even when the scale didn't indicate that I'd lost weight, I could tell by the way my clothes fit that my body was shrinking. After a few months, I could wear a belt. It had been nine years since I had worn a belt. My clothes got baggy, and I could actually feel a muscle in my thigh. I noticed that my watch was getting loose, my cheekbones were reappearing after many years in hiding, and I began to care about my appearance. My effort and commitment to exercise were working, and I could tell.

Your Turn

When is the best time for you to exercise and why? _____
_____
_____

What exercise do you think you might enjoy? _____
_____
_____

What physical benefits can you imagine would come from exercise? _____
_____
_____

Make Your Own Plan

First decide what time of day to exercise. It might be morning, as it was for me. Maybe you can squeeze in some time during your lunch hour. Or perhaps evening is best for you. When you exercise is a personal preference, but exercising in the morning gets the task out of the way. If you exercise first thing in the morning, you'll be less likely to skip a workout session because of an unscheduled afternoon meeting, a sick child, or a busy workload. Studies show that breaking up a thirty-minute exercise time into three ten-minute blocks is very effective. Believe me: The thirty minutes you take away from another activity will come back to you in the form of energy that you can spend on family, your career, or yourself!

Choose an exercise you will actually do and one that you are physically capable of doing. Buy an exercise DVD, borrow one from the library to see if you like that exercise, or watch a YouTube video of the exercise you are interested in. You can join a gym, walk, ride a bike, swim, or jog. There are many possibilities but only one outcome. If you commit to exercise, your health will improve. Most likely, you will start to feel better about yourself too.

Fitness Tips

Go with a Friend
Often, just knowing that your friend is counting on you to walk with her will get you out of bed and out the door.

Ask for a Trial Gym Membership
Many gyms offer short-term trial memberships. If you think you might like working out at a gym but are not sure about committing to a yearlong membership, stop by and ask about a trial membership.

Check out the Mall in Your Area
In all the cities we have lived in, the local mall opens early every weekday for the express purpose of allowing people to walk. Not only is the mall generally a safe place to walk, but it also takes any possibility of inclement weather out of the equation.

Check out Local Colleges and Universities
Many schools allow city residents to use their facilities for a small fee. Some colleges and universities even have pools.

Start Small
Don't head out the first day expecting to complete a marathon. By taking small but deliberate steps, you will see your fitness level improve without risking injury.

Drink Water
This advice is especially important if you are exercising outside in the heat or humidity. Stay well hydrated.

As You Improve, Up Your Intensity
Walk harder, longer, and faster as you are able.

Get the Right Shoes
If you are just beginning a walking program, take the time to visit a running store, where specially trained employees can select the best shoe for your feet and your activity level. It is worth the extra money to have a great pair of shoes!

Break It Up
If you do not have time for a thirty-minute block, exercise for three ten-minute intervals. Studies show that this method is almost as effective as one thirty-minute session. Don't let your schedule be an excuse.

Add in Strength Training
As your physical fitness increases and your weight comes down, add strength training into your routine. Light hand weights are inexpensive and readily available. You can also strengthen your muscles by performing planks and push-ups or by taking a Pilates class. Check with a friend who weight trains, take advantage of the trainers at your gym, or purchase a strength-training DVD.

Six Weeks Please

Commit to your exercise program for just six weeks at first. If you do not feel different after those six weeks, I'll be shocked. If your efforts haven't paid off, talk to your doctor. He or she might be able to recommend a more effective exercise regimen for you. The doctor might also perform tests to determine what might be preventing you from exercising successfully.

Use me as your role model. I wore awful clothes as I huffed and puffed uphill, hauled my lovely children with me, modified my exercise level when I needed to, and was never content to just stroll around the block. As I lost weight and as my fitness level improved, I strove to go faster than I had the week before. I worked my way up from walking at a snail's pace for a few minutes to speed walking around my neighborhood for forty-five minutes. Look how my body has changed. Your body can be whatever you want it to be. What do you want? Imagine it. Visually imagine yourself in the kind of shape you want to be in. Close your eyes and see yourself exercising at the weight you always dreamed of. If you can see yourself that way, you can be that way.

Congratulations on finishing another chapter! Meet you in the next section, where we will discuss how to incorporate the Fit to the Finish plan into your daily life.

PART III

November 1991 – 280 pounds

Conquer

to gain a victory
over; surmount;
master; overcome:

January 1991 – 260 pounds

October 1994 – 250 pounds

Implementing the Plan

Now that you have a good grasp of the three basic components of the Fit to the Finish plan, get ready to take hold of the plan and make it your own. In the following chapters, I discuss calories, hunger, habits, plateaus, holidays, and restaurant choices. Although I share many stories of my life as a fat woman, I also give you concrete suggestions on how to successfully navigate the often-difficult waters of weight loss. By the time you finish the section, you will have the tools to successfully venture on your weight-loss journey.

8

Good-bye Diets, Hello Lifestyle

Your lifestyle is a reflection of your belief system, your personal priorities, your family situation, and your work. As a person who struggled with her weight for many years, I can tell you that changing your lifestyle is possible and is a necessary part of weight maintenance. The word *lifestyle* as it relates to weight loss and weight maintenance refers to making consistently healthy food choices, controlling your calories, engaging in regular cardiovascular and strength-training workouts, and avoiding extreme swings in body weight. When I said good-bye to temporary diets that did not prepare me for long-term weight maintenance, I had to embrace a new lifestyle. In this chapter, I show you the importance of making a commitment to permanent lifestyle changes, and I show you how to do it.

Diet Crazy

Did you know that weight loss is a multibillion dollar industry? In 2007 Americans spent more than $58 billion on weight-loss-related products, according to the American Dietetic Association. How many of those billions of dollars were yours? Was your money put to good use, or do you look back and regret that you wasted money on programs, foods, or diet supplements that did not work?

When I first tried to lose weight, I spent my fair share of money on diet programs and foods, often borrowing money from other areas of the family budget. It seems ironic that we spend an incredible amount of money each year joining weight-loss centers and buying dieting supplements and nutrition aids, but more than 66 percent of Americans are overweight and nearly one-third are medically obese. On any given day, almost half of adult American women will tell you they are on a diet. Since this outlay of money does not translate to fewer Americans being obese or developing a healthy lifestyle, spending money on diet programs and supplements is obviously not the key to successful weight loss for most people. The National Weight Control Registry, of which I am a member, indicates that more than half the people who lose a significant amount of weight and maintain the loss do so without joining a commercial diet program.

Fast Results

Why are we getting bigger and bigger? And why is the diet industry such a moneymaker? One reason is that most of us are looking for a quick fix instead of a sustained lifestyle change. We have grown so accustomed to instant communication, fast food, microwaves, computers and tablets, Twitter, and flying cross-country in mere hours that we want and expect our weight-loss attempts to be equally fast.

I confess that I like things to happen fast. I don't like to stand in line at the store and will move from line to line in a fruitless attempt to get through faster. I click my computer mouse, shake the remote, turn the oven up to a higher temperature—anything to get things done faster. But rarely do these attempts work. The computer page doesn't load faster, the food burns, and shaking the remote doesn't do anything.

No matter what you read in advertisements or see on television, there is no quick fix for your weight problems. The only way to lose weight permanently and stop bouncing from one weight-loss program to another is to focus on one choice at a time. If you consider each meal, food, snack, and exercise workout as a means to create a new lifestyle, you will develop the strategies and willpower you need to make healthy food choices, and you will begin to see results.

Short-Sighted Diets

The basic problem with diets is the same, whether the diet recommends lots of protein or asks you to purchase specialty food from its local center or Web site. All diets seem to assume that simply losing weight is your ultimate goal, when in fact your ultimate goal as an overweight or obese person is to maintain a healthy weight throughout your life.

Some diets focus on only your food intake, without teaching and encouraging you to examine how you became overweight or obese in the first place. A lack of attention to the whys of your weight problem often leads to unintentionally repeating the same food habits and poor lifestyle choices that caused you to be overweight in the first place. This type of short-sighted diet assumes that just achieving weight loss will fix a poor lifestyle. As you continue throughout the book, I encourage you to do some soul searching to understand why you struggle with your weight.

Many short-sighted diet plans do not include exercise but focus only on calories. Often these programs provide you with food in prepackaged containers, thus carefully controlling your calorie intake. Missing from most of these programs is how to make a permanent change in how you cook, eat out, and shop for foods.

Diets that recommend eating mainly carbohydrates or mainly protein-rich foods might help you lose weight initially, but you might find it very difficult to continue eating from mostly one food group to the exclusion of others for the rest of your life. I know many people who lost impressive amounts of weight very quickly by following a high-protein diet but none who maintained their weight loss for more than a few months. One man lost more than 50 pounds in four months and regained the weight more quickly than he lost it. He came to me for advice. I was not surprised when he said that he assumed that once he lost the weight, he could just go back to eating as he had before his weight loss.

As you learn and apply the techniques in this book, you can move from a dieting mentality to a healthy lifestyle mentality and avoid the mental and physical anguish of regaining lost weight. When you combine that shift in thinking with a strategy for changing your lifestyle, you can maintain the weight you lose for years to come.

Remember, there is no quick fix or magic bullet. You did not gain weight overnight. You won't lose weight overnight. But it is possible to quickly change your lifestyle, and you can begin immediately. If you joined a plan in the past, or tried diet pills, you know what happens when the plan ends or the pill bottle is empty. You are left without help to complete your goal.

Hopefully, by this point we are all on the same page. Fit to the Finish is not a temporary diet. It's not a secret. It's not a magic bullet. It's a commonsense plan created by a stay-at-home mom of seven children who finally put it all together.

Your Turn

When you think of dieting, how do you feel? _____
_____
_____

Do you believe diets work? .... Yes ❑ No ❑

Why or why not? _____
_____

What do you have to change to permanently lose weight? _____
_____
_____

What will be hard about that? _____
_____
_____

Plan versus Diet

You probably noticed that I call Fit to the Finish a plan. When I think of the word *diet*, I think of a finite period of time, while a plan can be infinite. Plans carry on throughout time, while diets end when the program ends or your money runs out. Being fit and healthy requires making a permanent change in your eating and activity levels to match your new paradigm. Fit to the Finish is a lifestyle plan. No matter what your lifestyle currently is, the plan can help you maintain your healthy weight once you reach it. It does not matter if you work in an intense office job or stay home most of the day. All that matters is that you put your eating habits in proper perspective. Heed Ben Franklin's advice: "Eat to live, and not live to eat."

Diets do not often work, and permanent lifestyle changes can be hard to make. Why try then? Why put yourself through another attempt to get healthy when you may have failed in the past? If 95 percent of the people who lose weight on a particular diet gain it back, and a majority of people who start a diet program quit before reaching their goal weight, why don't we just quit trying? I think our brains are hardwired to succeed. That's why we want the instant results and work so hard to get ahead. Even though I failed over and over again with many diets, I thought about my weight all the time. What I never thought about was my lifestyle. I led the lifestyle of an unhealthy woman who did not care about her appearance, even though the opposite was true. Whether secretly eating entire boxes of cookies or munching through a bag of chips, I would think about how fat I was. I knew I was consuming an excessive number of calories, but I couldn't seem to stop. I didn't want to be a loser, but I was losing the battle for my weight because of my lifestyle.

I knew that some people lost large amounts of weight by dieting—I had seen their pictures on the wall of the meeting room where I was once again trying to achieve success. I had visual proof that a particular diet had worked for someone. Why would it not work for me? It did not work for me because instead of examining every area of my life for unhealthy lifestyle choices, I only thought about losing pounds.

Your Turn

How much weight would you like to lose? _____

_____

Can you do it? .... Yes ❑ No ❑

Why or why not? _____
_____
_____
_____

Making Lifestyle Changes

Here's a funny thing: when I needed to lose only 20 pounds, I thought that was a lot. I've come to realize that it doesn't matter how much weight you need to lose—it always seems like a lot. As my weight crept up, my confidence that I could get back to a regular size plummeted. Even so, somewhere in my heart I knew I could do it.

So if you checked no on the "Can you do it?" question above, go back and fix it. Make it yes—because you can do it. It took many years of starts and stops before I finally achieved long-term success. The key to my success was that I quit trying to diet and learned to adjust my lifestyle in a way that was sustainable. If I had given up, I'd probably be homebound now instead of enjoying an active life with my family.

How can you be confident that this time will be different? I'll tell you how: Do not think of the Fit to the Finish weight-loss plan as a temporary diet but rather as a lifelong way to achieve and maintain a healthy weight. Instead of thinking of yourself as dieting and therefore not able to eat like "regular" people (not that "regular" people eat very well), acknowledge that food is a difficult issue for you and that you are going to permanently change your lifestyle using the three prongs of the Fit to the Finish plan:

- Keeping the percentage of fat in your diet at 30 percent
- Consuming appropriate portion sizes
- Exercising regularly

Daily Food Choices

Think about your current food choices and how they impact your life. Do you make choices that you know are bad for you? Do you hide how much or what you eat from important people in your life?

I did. I knew no one was looking over my shoulder as I inhaled cookies, biscuits, chocolate candy, ice cream, and a host of other foods in excess. I was just fooling myself, although I thought I was fooling other people as well. After all, I was home alone with small children. Sometimes Rachel would say, "What are you eating Mommy?" as I attempted to quietly unwrap candy bars on the way home from the grocery story. I would lie and say, "Nothing." She knew, even in her little mind, that I was deceiving her. Every time I lied to my little girl, or told John that I didn't know what had happened to the ice cream that used to be in the freezer, I was not being transparent and honest about my true, unhealthy lifestyle.

Your Turn

Are there things you eat that you would rather no one know about? .... Yes ❑ No ❑

What are they? _____

_____

_____

Can you commit to not eating foods that you would be embarrassed to have someone else see you eat? _____

_____

_____

Making Better Choices

My journey to successful weight loss involved many choices. Some choices were easy, and some were hard. It was easy to say I was going to eat a healthier diet, but it was sometimes difficult to implement that choice. One thing I found immensely helpful was to picture someone I loved beside me as I went through my day, encouraging me to make good choices. Before I bought a bag of candy or pulled up to a drive-through window for a large order of French fries, I considered whether it was the best choice for me and whether I'd be embarrassed to have John or someone else I loved witness me eating it. Over time, making the healthy choice became something I was proud to share with John. As the number of healthy choices I made increased, my overall lifestyle changed for the better. I became accountable to myself for each choice I made, from choosing to exercise regularly to eating a balanced diet. I started each day anew and knew that each minute of the day, I had the chance to get closer to living the active lifestyle I desired.

As you reject the dieting philosophy and embrace a new lifestyle, remember that taking personal responsibility for your failures and successes is part of the weight-loss process.

Your Turn

Think of a time when you made a life change (for example, getting married, starting a new job, having a child, relocating). How did you handle it?

_____

_____

_____

Did the life change create any positive experiences? _____

_____

_____

Did it create any negative experiences? _____

_____

_____

How will committing to a new lifestyle of healthy eating and regular activity change your life for the better? _____

_____

_____

9

Responsibility: Owning It

Carol, a young woman in one of my classes, understood the need to reject temporary diets but found it hard to accept her own role in her weight problems. She and I were similar in that way, and I shared with her how I had learned to take responsibility for all my actions—both positive and negative. In taking responsibility for how you deal with food and exercise, you are moving one step closer to your goals.

One step in taking responsibility for your choices is to honestly acknowledge the weaknesses you have with food. To acknowledge your weakness surrounding food, look at why it is hard to change your lifestyle. You might have deeply ingrained habits from childhood, face challenging personal situations, or simply enjoy eating foods that are not good for you. Acknowledging the problem is often half the battle. Once you acknowledge that food is a struggle for you, the next step is learning how to win that battle.

If fessing up is the first step in gaining control over your food choices, and the second step is learning how to win the battle by consistently making healthy lifestyle choices, then putting aside any excuses or justifications is the third step. In this chapter, I encourage you to honestly examine whether you let justification or faulty excuses stand in the way of getting to and maintaining a healthy weight.

The Trigger Food Made Me Do It!

Trigger foods are foods that trigger an emotional or physical response, making it hard for us to resist them. My trigger food was chocolate. If someone had been watching me eat for several days, I would have been embarrassed. I would bake a pan of brownies and eat three-quarters of it before John came home for dinner. I would make two batches of chocolate chip cookies and eat one batch "on the side." I would buy a 1-pound bag of M&M's, give Rachel two or three candies (if I were feeling generous), and then proceed to eat the whole bag over the course of a day. Sometimes, if I had a lot of willpower, the bag would last for two days. I would squirrel it away on a high pantry shelf and throughout the day waddle over to the pantry, reach up high, and grab a few more of those colorful candies. Yes, I definitely had issues with chocolate.

Over the years, many people have shared with me their weakness for chips and crackers. They would open a chip bag, leave it on the counter, and throughout the afternoon eat the entire bag, just a few chips at a time. Some people are ice cream lovers; others just love all food and indulge with a passion. But for a lot of us, one particular food category is more tempting than others.

Your Turn

What is your favorite high-fat food? _____

_____

_____

How much of that food do you typically consume at one sitting? _____

_____

_____

_____

How many times a month do you typically indulge in that food? _____

_____

_____

_____

After you eat too much of that food, how do you feel physically? _____
_____
_____

How do you feel emotionally? _____
_____
_____

Have you ever hidden the fact that you have indulged in
this food from a significant person in your life?......................Yes ❑ No ❑

What were the circumstances? (Be honest.) _____
_____
_____

Why do you think this food is challenging for you to control? _____
_____
_____

The J Word—Justification

I tried to justify how much chocolate I ate by telling myself that I just could not resist the taste of chocolate. I tried to avoid taking personal responsibility for eating so much chocolate by blaming the food rather than blaming myself. But the chocolate did not magically appear in my pantry—I purchased the chocolate. Brownies did not make themselves—I prepared and ate them. Yes, chocolate was a trigger food for me, but I realized that I had to learn how to handle the trigger rather than give in to its lure.

While losing weight the final time, I developed strategies to deal with my strong emotional desire to eat chocolate. When I was tempted, I reminded myself that I could choose whether to purchase the chocolate or not. I reviewed my goals and acknowledged that eating large amounts of chocolate would likely push me further from my goals. Finally, I learned to fill the void by eating other sweet but healthy foods, such as fruit smoothies, strawberries, and sweetened yogurt.

For the first several weeks while following my plan, I decided I would not eat any chocolate. That was a huge step for me. But chocolate was a trigger food, and therefore too dangerous to have around. The very first test came quickly. My sweet husband, who liked to bring me food, was going on a business trip to California. His plane left very early, so he got up at four in the morning and rode to the airport with a friend. I vaguely remember him kissing me good-bye, and then I promptly fell back asleep. Imagine my surprise when I got up later that morning and saw a beautiful gift basket full of goodies sitting in the kitchen. He knew I disliked staying by myself, so he left treats to make me feel better.

In that basket were the most luscious, delectable treats I had seen in weeks. We had been married for ten years, so he knew what I liked. He had left an entire bag of Dove chocolate candy, a whole pound of Peanut M&M's, and several large pieces of gourmet chocolate. To John's credit, he also put in two bananas, several apples, and two magazines. I looked at that basket, lifted the heavy yellow M&M's bag in my hands, and then put it down. I prayed to God for self-control, as I was going to require a healthy dose of it. A few minutes later, the girls got up and squealed when they saw the basket. It took everything I had not to snap, "Get back—it's mine!" But I didn't. Instead, I took a deep breath, smiled sweetly at them, and said, "Look at the candy Daddy left for you girls."

"He left all that for us?"

"Yes, he did. Wasn't that nice of him?"

They were so excited and got even more excited when I handed them the bags of chocolate and said they could have a couple pieces each day. They were thrilled, and I felt that I had jumped a hurdle and taken responsibility for my own choices. I really wanted that chocolate, even though I knew it wouldn't fit into my weight-loss plan. John hadn't realized I was really serious about losing weight. He told me later that he didn't know how committed I had become to my plan and that he was sorry he had left me with so much temptation. In some ways it was good he left the candy for me. It showed me I could resist the desire to overindulge in a food that was hard for me to control, and it gave me confidence that I could do it again.

In my obese life, I justified eating food that was not on my plan because the food was free, someone had made me a special meal, I was tired, the food was low in fat, I deserved it, or any other number of excuses. When faced with that chocolate basket, I could have justified eating the chocolate treats by saying, "Well, John went to all that trouble to make the basket for me, so the least I could do is eat it so I don't hurt his feelings." I could have easily convinced myself it was okay to eat the chocolate, but for once I chose to break the cycle and stop making excuses. I took responsibility for myself and my weight. I encourage you to practice saying no to yourself and to see how it feels. I surmise that you will feel empowered. You will also realize that turning down a food you don't need is not the end of the world. Rather, it's the beginning of improving your control over food. Once I had achieved success that first time, I knew I could do it again.

When I was heavy, I often tried to justify an unhealthy food choice at the grocery store. I usually had a list as long as my arm, two children in the cart, and just thirty minutes to shop because of impending naps. So I'd fly through the store, throwing things in my cart with little or no regard for calories or fat. I felt incapable of not purchasing my trigger foods, and I never turned down the girls when they asked for candy or cookies. After all, they were small, and I could eat most of the bags without their knowledge.

I justified my purchases by convincing myself that I deserved those foods because I worked so hard. I also tried to convince myself that the brownies or Oreos were for John after a long day, not for me to feed my face.

Your Turn

What food items tempt you in the grocery store? _____
_____
_____

When buying an item, ask yourself:

Am I buying this food for my family or for myself? _____
_____
_____

Will I be tempted to consume this food if it's sitting in my pantry? ....Yes ❑ No ❑

If I eat too much of this food, will I feel guilty afterward?...........Yes ❑ No ❑

If the answer to the last question is yes, is that feeling of guilt worth the temporary pleasure the food offers? If you remember these questions as you shop, you will have the motivation to put those foods back. That act of putting unhealthy foods back on the shelf is the equivalent of taking responsibility for your weight.

Making the Hard Decisions

I wish I could tell you how many times I carried candy or cookies around a store, only to lay the package down somewhere right before I got to the cash register. I always felt good when I put the food back, although in the car on the way home I would think, *I can't believe I didn't buy any chocolate!* But I would quickly forget about the chocolate and was very proud of myself for resisting. It felt good to finally have some control over food. The self-control didn't come overnight, but by giving myself some strong parameters in the beginning, I experienced small successes, which eventually led to ultimate triumph.

These days, my seven children often ask for treats, and I sometimes buy them. But during my first year of weight loss, I suggested alternatives to the foods I liked too much. For instance, if the kids asked for chocolate graham crackers, I bought the honey version. This satisfied them and helped me avoid the temptation of having chocolate crackers in the house. By purchasing foods I did not like, I was able to reduce the temptation to overeat. As time went on and I became stronger and more aware of my needs versus my desires, I was able to buy danger foods without worrying that I would not be able to resist them.

As you go grocery shopping over the next weeks and months, think about the items you purchase. Determine whether you really need that bag of chips or that candy bar or whether you are trying to justify purchasing it.

Excuses, Excuses, Excuses

You've probably used some of the same excuses I used to avoid taking responsibility for your weight-loss problems. You likely also have an arsenal of reasons for why your past diets failed. I found it very easy to be dishonest with myself about my food choices but taking responsibility for myself and not making excuses for my failures were some of the most important parts of my eventual success.

Here I list six common excuses for diet failure and give you ideas about how to push those excuses aside and succeed.

My Diet Failed because It Was Too Hard to Follow

This was my favorite excuse. If a friend asked me what happened to my latest diet, I would say it was too hard to follow. This could mean anything from I didn't like the food I had to eat to the unfortunate fact that the diet required me to give up sweets. It was a good catch-all excuse that seemed to cover all the required bases. In reality, the diet wasn't too hard to follow. After all, most diets are pretty simple. In reality, I didn't want to diet anymore. I made the choice to quit following the diet's recommendations, and I justified it to myself by saying it was too hard. My friends probably got used to this excuse and came to expect it.

My Diet Failed because of a Holiday

As with most families, holidays are a big deal to us. John and I celebrate all holidays, major and minor, and celebrations usually revolve around food. Birthdays feature a cake, ice cream, and treats. Thanksgiving brings turkey, dressing, green bean casserole, apple pie, pumpkin pie, cheesecake, and nuts. At Christmastime come dozens of cookies, numerous parties, buffet lines, and office celebrations. Easter holds the promise of chocolate candy, glazed ham, deviled eggs, and cake. We celebrate the Fourth of July, Labor Day, and Memorial Day with enormous picnics, complete with a smorgasbord of food selections. And let us not forget one of my favorite holidays, Valentine's Day. Valentine's Day is all about the chocolate! From minor holidays to major anniversaries, we celebrate them all with food. Why is that? For us, we love to be together, and we love to eat. When I was dieting, it wasn't the holiday that caused the problem. The problem stemmed from my using the holiday as a built-in excuse for once again giving up.

My Diet Failed because It Was That Time of the Month

For female readers, this excuse may have some validity. Research shows that women in the latter half of their monthly cycle have a drop in serotonin levels, or the "feel-good" hormone. The levels drop when estrogen drops and progesterone increases. As your serotonin level decreases, you may find yourself craving chocolate or another comfort food, making it difficult to stick to your healthy eating plan. Therefore, you might have a true biological reason for those monthly chocolate cravings, but it's important to keep these types of cravings in perspective. Even though I didn't know about the science at the time, I used hormonal cravings as an excuse to stop my weight-loss attempts. But I didn't need to eat 16 ounces of Peanut M&M's followed by a bag of chips and some ice cream. I just liked having something to blame my problems on.

My Diet Failed because I Had to Go out of Town

Looking back, this was a lame excuse. What in the world did going out of town have to do with dieting? I understand it can be harder to control your food intake when you are not doing the cooking, but it's not impossible. You can always make the best choices from what is available. Traveling for a day or two certainly doesn't mean you have to quit your diet altogether. But you'd never know it by following my example when I was obese.

When I joined Weight Watchers for the eighty-second time (yes, you read that correctly) and lost several pounds, I told all my friends that *this time* I was finally going to get rid of all the excess pounds I was carrying around. But life got in the way, and summer rolled around. Off we went to visit John's mom. While driving up to the coast, I ate and drank the following:

- One bag of pretzels
- Two bags of Peanut M&M's
- A 32-ounce half-diet/half-regular Coke
- A Big Grab bag of Cheetos
- Six Oreo cookies

And that was just on the drive up. Something about packing the car, loading the kids, and leaving town made me want to overeat. Once we arrived at John's mother's house, the food fest really began in earnest. Cookies, chips, huge dinners, and new restaurant meals called my name, and I willingly answered. Every time my mother-in-law asked if I'd like something to eat, I said yes. The continual eating and complete lack of exercise meant that during that five-day vacation, I gained back the 6 pounds I had lost on Weight Watchers. And to make matters worse, I also lost any incentive for trying to complete my weight-loss journey. "Oh well," I reasoned, "I'm just meant to be fat."

Every vacation during my obese years unfolded the same way. Utter lack of planning, contempt for healthy food choices, and complete abandonment of any eating plan sabotaged my desire to lose weight and get fit.

My Diet Failed because I Didn't Like the Leader at the Weight Watchers Meeting

I used this excuse not only as a reason to quit my diets but also as a reason to not attend meetings at all. Weight Watchers holds more than one meeting per week. If you don't like one leader, you can just switch meetings. But instead of switching meetings, I just quit going. I reasoned that if I didn't care for one leader, I probably wouldn't like any of them.

My Diet Failed because I Had Out-of-Town Company

I used this excuse frequently, as it was common for us to have houseguests. I reasoned that they wouldn't want to eat low-fat rabbit food, so I always broke out my favorite high-fat recipes when company came to call.

My Diet Failed because I Hit a Plateau

I distinctly remember my first official diet. In my first year of marriage, I gained about 15 pounds. I was still average size but was pleasingly plump. I wasn't happy being plump, so I joined Weight Watchers during my second year of marriage. I consistently attended meetings and did well. My goal was to lose 15 to 20 pounds. After ten weeks, I had lost about 13 pounds. Then I stopped losing weight. Week 11 came and went—no weight loss. Week 12 came full of hope and anticipation, but then I stepped on the scale—no weight loss. Week 13 came, and with great apprehension I stepped on the scale—only to be confronted with no weight loss! That was it. I quit. Did I ask anyone for advice? No. Did I read a book, try to exercise, cut back more on my eating? No. Did I keep going to meetings?

No. I quit and told everyone that Weight Watchers just wasn't working for me anymore. I reasoned my body must be happy at my new weight and therefore I should quit.

Your Turn

Have you used excuses to avoid taking responsibility for
your weight-loss failures?.. Yes ❏ No ❏

List one or two excuses you have used: _____

_____

_____

Do you accept that taking responsibility for your actions
can do away with the need for excuses? .... Yes ❏ No ❏

Shedding the "It's Not My Fault" Mentality

Getting rid of excuses leaves only you. Gone is the facade of diets not working because of invalid excuses. Removed forever is the ability to justify poor choices. Trigger foods will lose their pull when you acknowledge your weaknesses and develop strategies to deal correctly with those foods.

You might find it harsh when I say you must shed the "it's not my fault" mentality, but this is vital to long-term success. Unless you have a metabolic disorder or some other medical component to your weight problem, the fault is yours—just like my problem was mine. That was hard to accept, but in a sense it was very freeing.

By admitting my own culpability in my weight problems, I also freed myself up to make positive changes. Each time I put aside an excuse or refused to justify a poor choice, it was like giving myself a gold star. The more imaginary gold stars I accumulated, the stronger I got. You will find that accepting responsibility for yourself increases your confidence in your ability to make good choices and to move your life in the direction you desire.

10

Calorie Awareness

Fit to the Finish does not focus on counting calories or fat grams. Instead, the plan focuses on the percentage of fat in your diet, perfecting portion control, and increasing your commitment to exercise. However, I do believe that being aware of the calorie and fat content in foods is an important piece of any successful diet and weight-maintenance plan. Once you become educated on approximately how many calories you need to maintain a healthy weight, you will have one more tool to guide you on your lifelong journey.

How Many Calories Do You Need?

How many calories you need is dependent on many factors, such as your age, gender, activity level, and weight goals. To determine the approximate number of calories you need to *maintain* your weight, with no exercise, multiply your weight by 10 (if you are a woman) or by 11 (if you are a man). That number is your resting calorie estimate. Then, using the chart below, multiply your resting calorie estimate by your activity level multiplier.

Activity Level	Multiplier
Sedentary (desk job; no exercise)	1.2
Light activity (light exercise 2–3 days per week)	1.375
Moderate activity (moderate exercise 3–5 days per week)	1.55
Heavy activity (heavy exercise every day)	1.725
Super activity (heavy athletics or hard labor)	1.9

A 150-pound woman, for example, would multiply her weight by 10 to get a resting calorie level of 1,500. If she were lightly active, she would then multiply 1,500 by 1.375 to get 2,063. Therefore, she needs approximately 2,000 calories per day to maintain her weight at her current activity level.

A 200-pound man would multiply his weight by 11 to get a resting calorie estimate of 2,200. If he were lightly active, he'd then multiply 2,200 by 1.375 to get 3,025. So he needs approximately 3,000 calories to maintain his weight at his current activity level.

Your Turn

In this exercise, you will perform two different calculations: one for your current weight and one for your desired weight.

For Women

Current weight: _____ × 10 = _____ (resting calorie requirement)

Resting calorie requirement: _____ × activity level multiplier = _____ (daily calories needed to maintain current weight)

Desired weight: _____ × 10 = _____ (resting calorie requirement)

Resting calorie requirement: _____ × activity level multiplier = _____ (daily calories needed to maintain desired weight)

For Men

Current weight: _____ × 11 = _____ (resting calorie requirement)

Resting calorie requirement: _____ × activity level multiplier = _____ (daily calories needed to maintain current weight)

Desired weight: _____ × 11 = _____ (resting calorie requirement)

Resting calorie requirement: _____ × activity level multiplier = _____ (daily calories needed to maintain desired weight)

The main point of this exercise is to emphasize that your calorie needs will change as you lose weight. As you increase your activity level, you will expend more energy (burn more calories), and your calorie needs will increase. But as you lose weight, you will need to adjust your calories downward (or increase your activity level). If you do not adjust your calorie consumption or your activity level, your weight loss will stall, and you will end up on a plateau.

Fat Grams and the Fat Percentage Formula

The occasional nutrition labels, particularly those from other countries, show only fat grams and not calories from fat. It's important to be able to convert fat grams to calories and vice versa. It's also helpful to know how many total fat calories and fat grams you can consume in a day.

Now that you know approximately how many calories you should be eating per day, the next step is to determine how many of those calories can be derived from fat. To do this, take the number of calories you need per day to maintain your current weight and multiply it by .30, or 30 percent.

The resulting number looks large, doesn't it? In our example above, the lightly active woman who weighs 150 pounds and needs to eat approximately 2,000 calories per day can have 600 of her calories from fat (2000 x .30 = 600). To determine how many fat grams that equals, divide 600 by 9 (the number of calories per fat gram). That calculation gives you 67. So she can have 67 fat grams per day, at most.

Your Turn

Calculate the number of fat grams you can have per day at your current weight:

Current resting calorie requirement: _____ × .30 = _____
(calories from fat per day)

Calories from fat per day _____ ÷ 9 = _____
(number of fat grams per day)

Calculate the number of fat grams you can have per day at your desired weight:

Desired resting calorie requirement: _____ × .30 = _____
(calories from fat per day)

Calories from fat per day _____ ÷ 9 = _____
(number of fat grams per day)

These calculations give you the total number of fat grams you can have per day and still achieve a total fat percentage under 30 percent. You might wonder why I had you calculate both your current weight and your desired weight requirements. First of all, the numbers will change as you lose weight. More important, if you attune your calorie intake to your desired weight rather than your current weight, you are guaranteed to lose weight. Fabulous!

The Ins and Outs of Calorie Counting and the Importance of a Target Calorie Count

I tried counting calories during one of my many weight-loss attempts. One day while standing in line at the grocery store, I bought a little booklet that listed the calorie content of a large variety of foods. Knowing me, I probably had a cart full of high-fat foods at that very moment. Nonetheless, during that calorie-counting diet, I was religious about writing down the number of calories I consumed for one week. Each and every time I ate something, I calculated the number of calories, wrote it down in my booklet, and kept a running total of the calories I had consumed for the day. At that time, my calorie goal was 1,540.

During that first week, I lost 5 pounds and was very proud of myself. During week 2, I mostly followed my booklet plan and wrote down about 80 percent of what I ate. That week I lost 2 pounds. The third week, because I was doing so well on the diet and already knew how many calories I was eating, I wrote in my booklet only about 50 percent of the time. That week I gained 1 pound. That weight gain made me angry, so I decided to "get back" at the little booklet. I stopped writing anything down, and within three weeks I had gained back 10 pounds. As I slowly stopped keeping track of my food intake, I also stopped losing weight and began to gain it. Why? Once I stopped writing in the booklet, I quickly reverted to my old eating habits, and the result was weight gain.

Although I did not count calories or fat grams when I was losing weight the last time, I was aware of my calorie and fat needs. When I hit the occasional plateau, I monitored my calorie and fat intake to make certain I was not eating too little or too much.

One such plateau occurred when I had been on my weight-loss journey for almost a year, and I was getting close to where I wanted to be. At that point, I probably had another 15 pounds to lose.

Several weeks went by with no weight loss, but instead of getting frustrated, as I normally would have, I got serious. I began to calculate how many calories I needed to eat for my desired weight. I kept a food journal for about a week and realized right away that I was eating a few more calories, and thus more fat, than I needed. I adjusted my calorie level down slightly, ramped up my activity level, and saw the scale move again. I was careful not to reduce my calories below 1,200 a day, as I wanted to keep my energy level high, nourish my body adequately, and avoid feeling extreme hunger.

If I hadn't known what my target calorie range was, I would have found it difficult to accurately assess the situation.

How Our Bodies Process Food

A calorie is a unit of energy, and anything that contains energy has calories. For our purposes, though, we'll look at calories only in relation to food. We use energy in all we do, from sleeping to running to eating. We get our energy from the food we consume. Without food and beverages we wouldn't have the energy to function properly.

The number of calories in food is a measure of how much potential energy the food contains. Food can be divided into three categories: carbohydrates, protein, and fat. These three categories are the foundation of the food we need to survive and thrive. The following chart shows how many calories each type of food contains:

Caloric Breakdown

1 g carbohydrates: 4 calories
1 g protein: 4 calories
1 g fat: 9 calories

Our bodies burn the calories in our food by using enzymes to break the carbohydrates into glucose and other sugars, the fats into glycerol and fatty acids, and the proteins into amino acids. These substances then move through the bloodstream to our cells, where they are used for a variety of processes. Your body uses some of the energy from the foods you eat immediately for energy, while other compounds are stored in your body tissues, such as your muscles, fat, and liver. Your metabolism functions with a dual-role. On one hand, your body stores energy from foods you eat and uses the nutrients to build up body tissues and grow new cells. This process is called anabolism. The other side of the metabolic coin, catabolism, is the mechanism that allows your body to release the massive amounts of energy you need to keep your body warm, to walk or run, to perform your daily activities, and to remove waste from your body.

Calories, Fat and Exercise

Logically, if you take in more calories than your body needs, you gain fat. Conversely, if you take in fewer calories than your body needs, you lose fat. Because your body stores extra calories for future need, when you burn more calories than you take in, the body will convert stored fat into energy to make up for the deficit.

Exercise can move your weight loss from one level to the next. Exercise raises your metabolic rate, which is the number of calories you use each day for all your activities. When you exercise, your metabolic rate increases and stays elevated for about two hours after you've stopped exercising. During that time, your increased metabolic rate continues to help your body burn calories.

Is a Calorie a Calorie?

Does it matter what you eat if all calories are processed through your body the same way? Technically—for weight loss—no. A calorie is a calorie, and as long as you burn off what you are eating, you will maintain your weight. A lot of us are simply taking in more calories than we burn, resulting in weight gain. So if one calorie is basically the same as another calorie, then you can just eat candy and junk food as long as you don't eat too many calories of those bad foods, right? No. The goal of any good weight-loss plan, including Fit to the Finish, is not only to lose weight but to improve your health and fitness level.

A friend once told me a very entertaining story about her husband's family. When she and her husband were dating, he was very thin but always sick. He constantly had colds, complained about being tired, and often caught whatever virus was going around school. She never asked him about his dietary habits, which included a lot of junk food and few vegetables. After all, they were teenagers.

They dated throughout college and got married soon after graduation. Once they were married and she began preparing his meals, he stopped getting sick. He finally realized that years of junk food, inactivity, and little to no vegetables had most likely weakened his immune system and zapped his energy. She told me that in the ten years of their marriage, he had gotten sick only once. Healthy food is powerful food.

To maintain a certain weight or to lose weight in a healthy, nutritionally sound way, you must go beyond just keeping track of calories or fat grams. Where your calories come from makes a big difference in how you feel and in how well your body functions. We know that complex carbohydrates (such as whole grains, beans, starchy vegetables) and that lean proteins (such as low-fat dairy, skinless chicken, or fish) are more healthful than foods high in saturated or trans fat, so it stands to reason that more of our calorie intake should come from the nutritionally superior calories. We do need some fat in our diets, but I promise you, most Americans have no problem taking in enough fat. If you take in 2,000 calories a day and limit calories from fat to 30 percent, for a maximum of 600 calories from fat, or 67 grams of fat per day, you're far from depriving yourself.

Here are some calorie and fat contents of common foods. The numbers might surprise you:

Food	Serving Size	Calories	Fat Grams	Calories from Fat	Percent from Fat
Canola oil	1 tbsp	120	14	120	100
Peanut butter	2 tbsp	190	16	130	68
Cheddar cheese	1 oz	114	9.4	85	75
Granola	1/2 c	145	5	45	31
Chocolate syrup	2 tbsp	100	0	0	0
Sugar	1 c	774	0	0	0
Coca-Cola	1 can	140	0	0	0

Well, that's interesting, isn't it? This chart is a great illustration of why it can be unhealthy to just count calories or fat grams. Notice that chocolate syrup, sugar, and Coca-Cola are all fat free but certainly not calorie free. If you were to base a diet plan on just counting fat grams, it would still be easy to eat too many calories. It can be confusing and difficult to decide what and how much to eat.

When I was overweight, I ate more than enough calories to keep me going, but I ate the wrong types of food, so I didn't have a lot of energy. And to make matters worse, it was tiring to move all my fat around. If you eat nutritionally empty calories, such as sugar-filled sweets or baked chips, you are doing your body a disservice. Those foods have few energy-giving complex carbohydrates, contain the wrong types of fat, and take up calorie space in your diet that you should be filling with nutritionally dense foods such as fruits, vegetables, low-fat dairy, and lean protein.

Calories are very important to our bodies, and we need a certain amount of fat to keep our bodies healthy, so why not count calories? Why not count fat grams? Why not do both? If you know how many calories your body needs to run efficiently, you could keep track of your calories, exercise consistently, and be done with it. If you do this and don't cheat on portion sizes, then you will likely lose weight.

Some people in my Fit to the Finish classes were very disciplined and had some success with calorie counting on previous diets. But even ultra-disciplined people eventually tire of calorie counting and gain some or all of their weight back. My suggestion is, rather than count calories, develop an *awareness* of calories.

Your Turn

Based on your best guess, how many calories do you normally consume per day? _____
_____
_____

What did you have for dinner last night? _____
_____

How many calories and fat grams do you guess your dinner had? _____
_____

According to calculations performed at the beginning of this chapter, how many calories should you be eating? _____
_____

Do you admit that you are probably eating more calories
per day than you should? .... Yes ❑ No ❑

Why do you think you are eating more than you should? _____
_____
_____

Do you ever say this to yourself: It's not that I eat too
many calories; I have a slow metabolism? .... Yes ❑ No ❑

On what do you base your response? _____
_____
_____

Facing the Truth

Without careful calculation, it is hard to know the actual number of calories you eat during the day. But if you're honest with yourself, you intuitively know whether you are consuming the proper number of calories. For a long time, I was in denial as to the actual amount of food I was eating. Numerous people have told me funny and sad stories about their eating habits. They have admitted eating cartons of ice cream, going to two different fast-food restaurants at their lunch hour, inhaling chocolate by the pound, and eating all the leftovers from a family meal when no one was looking. At the same time, they often complained to anyone who would listen that they just could not lose weight! I think these people knew in their hearts and innermost being that they were eating too many calories but could not bring themselves to admit it. When I coach people who want to lose weight, I find that one of the hardest sessions is when people come to terms with how many calories they were eating and how that choice negatively affected their lives.

Whether you count calories regularly is your decision. If you do, see appendix E for a calorie-counting worksheet. You can photocopy the page and use it to keep track of your calories.

11

What Are You Hungry For?

The hardest part of losing weight before my last, successful attempt wasn't lack of knowledge or understanding but rather the never-ending battle in my mind. Although I understood that eating candy for breakfast was not healthy or good for my waistline, I still found it hard to resist consuming a candy bar when I woke up. I believed the medical professionals who said that exercise was important, but I could not convince myself that getting off the couch and taking a walk would make a difference in my life. Over the years, a lot of people have asked me, "Diane, don't you think it's an emotional battle—the whole weight issue?" I agree that we put on weight and struggle to take it off partly due to emotional eating, but we also put on weight and have trouble losing it because of the food choices we make. The physical reality of weight management is an energy imbalance. We are eating more calories than we are burning. The emotional reality of weight management is an emotional imbalance. We eat when we are not physically hungry but when we are trying to fill an emotional need.

Appetite versus Hunger

True physical hunger is an unmistakable feeling. It occurs when your body physically signals to you that it needs nourishment. Contractions of your stomach muscles signal an increase in hunger. Blood glucose levels also tell your stomach to send the "hungry" signal to your brain.

Appetite is different from hunger. Appetite is based on emotion, which means your appetite might increase whether you are hungry or not. For example, a TV advertisement for your favorite dessert or favorite restaurant can evoke an emotional response in you. You might unconsciously or consciously begin to think, *I want that now.* If you are like me, you might find it difficult to get those advertising images out of your head. Before I started losing weight using Fit to the Finish, emotions would drive me to get up and make a dessert or to call John to schedule a lunch or dinner date at the advertised restaurant.

Feeling full, on the other hand, involves the disappearance of hunger symptoms after consuming food. However, the feeling of fullness can take several minutes to reach the brain, which is why dieticians and nutritionists recommend you stop eating before you reach the point of total fullness.

What occurs when you are hungry? What physical sensations do you experience? How do these sensations relate to what you actually eat? When I answered these questions, I gave two very different sets of answers, from two different points in my life. When I was overweight, I answered the first question like this: "I can't remember the last time I felt true hunger." As for the second question, I was unable to accurately describe the physical sensation of hunger because it had been so long since I'd felt it.

These days, as an average-size person, I experience hunger at the appropriate times. I am usually hungry when I wake up in the morning, particularly if I didn't eat too much at dinner the night before. I occasionally experience hunger during the day. I know I'm hungry because my stomach feels empty and sometimes makes embarrassing noises.

Your Turn

When was the last time you felt true physical hunger? _____
_____

Describe the circumstances: _____
_____

Describe the physical sensation: _____
_____

Hunger Avoidance

If you're overeating, chances are you're avoiding hunger. Why do you think you avoid hunger? What is so bad about being a little bit hungry? What is it that makes us run to food for comfort? I'm not a psychologist, so I can speak only from my personal experience and from the experiences of those who have shared their stories with me. A lot of us abuse food. I know that's a strong statement, but it's true. The definition of abuse is "to use wrongly." If you've read my story, I think you'll agree that I abused food.

If you struggle with your weight and if your weight problem is due to eating too much food, then logically speaking, you are not using food as it was intended. When you overeat, you are not only abusing food. You are also damaging your body and your spirit. It's a hard cycle to break.

Below is a list of possible reasons for eating when you're not physically hungry. The list comes partly from my own personal experience and partly from the very honest people I've taught over the years. Do any of these reasons resonate with you?

Reasons for Eating When You're Not Hungry

Control	Nerves	Depression
Stress	Happiness	Inadequacy
Loneliness	Anger	Excitement
Fear	Frustration	Anxiousness
Boredom	Sadness	Habit

Your Turn

Which of these reasons jump out at you? _____
_____

Do you have any additional reasons for eating when you're not hungry?
_____
_____

What is your first response when you do feel hunger? _____
_____
_____
_____

Food Gave Me a Feeling of Control

I've spent a lot of time thinking about hunger and why I abused food for so many years. I believe my biggest reason was a desire for control. I grew up in a difficult adoptive home, in which compliance was expected and disobedience in any form was not tolerated. I was obedient as a child and a pretty cooperative teenager, but it didn't make a difference. No matter what I did, it wasn't good enough for my parents. They loved me the best they knew how, but I still had a difficult childhood.

We all have issues, either from the past or present, that affect us in a variety of ways. Instead of using drugs or alcohol to escape or cope, I used food. Food was the one thing my parents couldn't control. My mom couldn't stop me from eating when I was away from home. Even at home, she couldn't always prevent me from overeating. I developed the habit of hiding food. When I went on an errand, I would swing by the drugstore or the grocery store and buy something sweet. Upon arriving home, I would stuff the candy in my purse and nonchalantly go to my room. Once there, I would unpack my stash and hide it in various places. (The back of my closet was a favorite location.) Whenever I needed some fortification, I would run to my room. I felt powerful and in control when I overate, almost as if I were getting back at someone for hurting me. I see now that the only person I was hurting was myself. I began a long cycle of using food inappropriately.

Your Turn

What, besides nourishment, do you use food for? _____
_____
_____
_____

What emotions cause you to head for the pantry or the drive-through window? _____

_____

_____

What past or current hurts make you want to overeat? _____

_____

_____

_____

Do certain foods bring back good memories?......................... Yes ❏ No ❏

Have you ever used food to assert your independence?.......... Yes ❏ No ❏

Did your parents or loved ones use food as a soother
for hurt feelings? .... Yes ❏ No ❏

Do you ever use food to assert yourself or to punish others? .. Yes ❏ No ❏

If you answered yes, why do you think you do this? _____

_____

_____

_____

Admitting Your Role

My situation was complicated, and yours may be as well. I had a difficult childhood, but I don't blame my overeating on my upbringing. How we react as adults is our responsibility. I was the one overeating. I was the one hiding food. I was the one who ate myself to morbid obesity.

Let's face it, you don't get to be obese without eating too much food—unless you have a medical condition or genetic abnormality that causes weight gain. No one was there shoving food at me. I did it to myself. Over the years, many situations sent me running to my favorite source of comfort—food. When I got stressed at work, I ate. When I had a lot of things on my schedule, I ate. When I was really happy, I ate. When I got nervous, I ate.

My cycle of overeating continued through college and into married life. When John and I married, I still found myself secreting food away. It was crazy, because John certainly never judged me for what I ate. In fact, he was usually right there stuffing his face with me. Once I finally began to change a lifetime of eating habits, I realized I needed to examine why I was doing what I was doing. I knew on some level it was for control and to have something to keep me busy all the time. I also reacted to stress, boredom, anxiety, and excitement by eating. In other words, I used almost any emotion as a reason to eat, because food was a source of comfort for me.

Your Turn

What emotions play into your eating habits? _____

_____

_____

_____

What situations cause you to overeat? _____

_____

_____

_____

What conclusions can you draw from these answers? _____

_____

_____

_____

As you examine your eating habits, you learn to put the bad habits aside and to replace them with new, healthy habits. I needed to put my emotional reactions from the past behind me and reach forward to the positive life I wanted to live. I'm not saying this battle is easy, but it is winnable. Once you know the causes of your poor eating habits, you can watch out for the danger signals.

Using Food to Fill a Void

In the old days, I could eat a large amount of food in a short period of time. I remember one incident in particular. It was after Rachel was born. I was still in the new mother adjustment period. After a year as a stay-at-home mom, I felt lonely much of the time. A lot of my friends were working and hadn't yet begun their families. Loneliness was a huge trigger for me. That day in 1991, I was sitting around the house feeling sorry for myself. The television was quietly humming in the background, and my mind told me to eat. I went to the food cabinet and started foraging. First I ate what was left in a box of cheese crackers, then I finished off the chips, and after that I needed something sweet. But I had finished off the ice cream the night before, and John had eaten the cookies. There was nothing sweet in the house.

Rachel was sleeping, and even in my desperation for a sweet treat, I wasn't about to wake her and head to the grocery store. I did the next best thing. I broke out my favorite cookbook, looked for the cookie recipe that made the largest batch, and began baking. I immediately felt my spirits rise as the chocolate dough began to form in the mixing bowl. I could almost taste the cookies, even though they hadn't even gone into the oven yet. Once the batter was in the oven, I stood in front of the appliance, willing the dough to cook faster. The minute the cookies were done, I pulled them out of the oven, removed them from the cookie sheet, and ate the entire first batch. It probably took me less than five or six minutes to eat two dozen cookies. I'm not even sure I tasted them. By the time Rachel woke up, I had eaten about three dozen chocolate cookies. The sad thing was—I was still hungry, but not for food.

Learning to recognize hunger and learning not to fear it are important steps in conquering the overeating cycle. I was afraid to be hungry and hadn't experienced true hunger for years. Consequently, when I first started changing my eating habits, hunger was an unfamiliar feeling.

Your Turn

How often are you hungry? _____

_____

Are you hungry more now than before you started
the Fit to the Finish Plan? .... Yes ❏ No ❏

What time of day are you likely to experience the most intense hunger?

_____

_____

What is the most common food you reach for at that time? _____

_____

_____

Why that particular food? _____

_____

_____

Strange Sensations

If you have started to change your eating habits, you've probably experienced some hunger sensations. This is good! I'm not advocating starving yourself or waiting until you are ravenous to eat, but a little bit of hunger sends a cue to your brain that your body needs nourishment.

When I was obese, I didn't even wake up hungry because after dinner John and I would continue snacking right up until bedtime. It was like "Dinner—Round Two!" We would make a pan of tortilla chips and cheese to eat while we were watching television and then forage in the pantry or the refrigerator for something sweet to finish off the night. In the morning when I woke up, the food parade would begin again. It didn't wrap up until after the sun went down.

Hunger is a normal sensation. Be proud that you are eating healthy portions and that you are beginning to allow your body to function as intended. If you are overweight, you are eating more food than your body can process efficiently. It is nearly impossible to feel full all the time while watching your caloric intake. As you are reducing your calorie count, you will feel hungry on occasion. It's okay.

I still remember the first time I woke up hungry. I had been following my plan for a couple of days, and one of the first habits I worked on breaking was eating after dinner. After a couple of nights of no snacking, I started waking up hungry. It was such a strange feeling to be hungry before 10:00 a.m. Before I started losing weight, I'd wake up full and proceed to eat all kinds of sweets in the morning. Donuts, brownies, candy—whatever was around the house. Instead, I made a concerted effort to make healthy breakfast choices, such as oatmeal, cereal, or fruit. I was amazed at the difference in how I felt. I felt energized, fortified, and ready for the day. I practiced paying attention to the feeling of hunger, listening to the signals my body naturally gave me. True physical hunger meant it was time to eat something nutritious.

What to Do When Hunger Strikes

There are different strategies for handling true hunger and emotional hunger. What should you do when you aren't really hungry but feel the emotional need to grab something to eat? If you have had a meal recently yet find yourself drifting toward the food cupboard, I want you to do three things: STOP. EVALUATE. WAIT.

STOP before you get to the pantry, the snack drawer, or the vending machines at work. STOP before you pull through your favorite fast-food drive-through. STOP before you reach for the candy dish in your friend's office. If you can put on the brakes at this point, you will give yourself the opportunity to make a wise choice. The more wise choices you put in your bank, the more confidence you develop. The more confidence you develop, the better long-term success you will have.

Now that you have stopped, it is time to evaluate. EVALUATE: What are you hungry for? EVALUATE: When was the last time you ate? EVALUATE: What do you really need right now? If you have recently eaten a meal or a good snack, then most likely food is not what you need. This is the hard part. What need is it that you are looking to fulfill? If it's not food, then what?

Finally, WAIT. Wait for fifteen minutes before you make any food decision. Let's assume that you really do feel hunger, even though you ate recently. You know you shouldn't still be hungry, so you decide to wait fifteen minutes and then reevaluate. This is not easy. It is very difficult to break the cycle of instant gratification—but it is definitely possible.

While you are letting your fifteen minutes go by, try moving your body to see if that motivates you to make wiser choices. If you are at the office, take a walk down the hallway, walk up and down a flight of stairs, or unobtrusively do some leg lifts while sitting in your office chair. If after fifteen minutes you are still hungry, even though according to the clock you shouldn't be, eat one portion of a healthy snack.

Let's set up a probable scenario: You ate a decent breakfast, had a healthy snack, and made it through lunch uneventfully. It's been only one hour since lunch ended, and your boss has just given you a huge assignment, which is due by the end of the day. What's your first thought? EAT! But, good for you, you've stopped in your tracks and decided to think before you eat. Now you are in the evaluation and waiting period.

Logically, you know you shouldn't be hungry. After all, you've just finished lunch. Let's think about what you were doing when you jumped up from your chair to head for the break room to answer the call of the vending machines.

Your first response when your boss gave you the assignment was to jump to food. But that's not really what you needed right then, was it? What you really needed was some stress relief. The only way to alleviate that particular stress is to finish the job, delegate the job to someone else, or get some help. Eating is not going alleviate that stress or get the assignment done.

For me, as a stay-at-home mom, eating triggers manifested themselves in a different form. If one of the children was sick, instead of just focusing on comforting her, I would alternate between comforting her and feeding myself. If we experienced difficult financial situations, then food was my solution. In fact, even being bored at home with small children was enough of a reason for me to eat.

Many times when the children were napping or off playing together, I didn't have anything to do. I'd wander around the house, in search of something to keep me busy. Instead of doing something productive, nine times out of ten I'd end up eating or baking. Oftentimes, the trigger that caused me to overeat was any type of stress or boredom.

Recognition of your own personal eating triggers is important, because if you can start to recognize bad habits when they arise, you can begin to break those habits.

Your Turn

When you start bingeing or overeating, what are you really hungry for?

_____

_____

What situations cause you to run for food? _____

_____

_____

Can you stop the situations from occurring? ....Yes ❏ No ❏

If you can't, what can you do to replace food as the first choice for stress relief?

_____

_____

_____

Recognition Is Key

Anytime I was nervous, bored, or stressed, it was as if an autopilot switch kicked on. I remember one time we were expecting out-of-town guests. They were due to arrive in a few hours. I was busy cleaning bathrooms, dusting furniture, pulling huge weeds out of planters, and eating my way through a bag of Double Stuf Oreos. Every time I walked through the kitchen, I'd grab another cookie or two. Crunch, munch, swallow, yum. One down, twenty-five to go. Each time I ate one, I told myself, _That's the last one_. But every time I saw the bag again, I'd eat more. By four in the afternoon, the house was almost ready for company. The furniture was dusted, the bathrooms were sparkling, but the floor was littered with Oreo crumbs where I had left a trail, like Hansel and Gretel, as I moved through the house munching through the entire bag of Oreos.

You would think that after gaining weight year after year, I would have begun to see a pattern to my eating habits. But I honestly didn't. I knew I was eating too much food on a daily basis, but I never evaluated why. I just attributed my excessive food intake to a lack of willpower. I couldn't recognize my problem, even though I sincerely desired to lose weight. Finally, through some careful introspection and by making conscious decisions to change poor habits, I understood the why and eventually lost the weight.

If you don't give in to your hunger immediately, it will go away and come back at a more appropriate time. Hunger is a real sensation, and eating cues are real. However, your emotions can also impact your desire to eat. Learning to tell the difference between emotional hunger and physical hunger by training yourself to stop, evaluate, and wait helps you distinguish between the two.

We've all heard it before: Eat when you are hungry; stop when you are full. That's what I'm advocating here, but with some steps built in to help you succeed. If you can use the three-step approach—stop, evaluate, and wait—you will find over time that you make the best choice more and more often.

Advanced Planning

Planning what you will eat when you are truly hungry between meals makes it less likely that you will grab the first food your hand touches in the pantry or make an unwise choice at your office vending machine. The truth is, as long as you make a wise choice, you can have whatever you want. Eat your chosen food and enjoy it guilt-free, knowing you were truly experiencing physical hunger and not trying to satisfy an emotional need.

Choose foods that will fill you up. Here are some good ideas:

Bread, Cereal, Rice and Pasta
Choose breads and cereals with a high-fiber content. Whole-grain breads, brown rice, and whole-grain pasta and cereals are good choices. When you eat rice or pasta, choose brown or wild rice over white rice and whole-wheat pasta instead of pasta made with white flour. Avoid small items, such as crackers and pretzels, as these are easy to eat in large quantities and are usually high in sodium.

Fruits and Vegetables
Almost all vegetables are low in calories and give you a decent amount of filling fiber. Although a snack of 2 cups of chopped carrots will give you fewer than 70 calories, you will likely be full before you start on the second cup. Limit your vegetable intake for snacking to one standard

serving, such as 1 cup of raw vegetables. The reason for limiting your intake is not because of the calorie content but to practice eating one serving or portion at a time. Fruits are also good choices. Limit your fruit servings to one piece of whole fruit or 1 cup of chopped fruit to avoid consuming too many calories from fruit. After all, a single large banana has more than 100 calories.

Milk, Yogurt and Cheese

These foods are good for you because they give you protein and calcium. However, the full-fat versions have more calories and fat than the reduced-fat or fat-free versions. Save yourself calories and consume less fat by choosing the healthier options of these foods.

Soups

Soup is a wonderful way to fill up. Just avoid cream-based soups, as they usually have a high fat content. If you purchase canned soups, be certain to watch the sodium content, as it can be extraordinarily high.

Beverages

It's a good idea to drink six to eight glasses of water each day. You may find, as I did, that when you stay adequately hydrated, you are less hungry. In fact, one of my first steps in avoiding unnecessary snacking was to make a cup of herbal tea. That often helped fill me up until my next meal. You can drink coffee, tea, or other low-calorie drinks in addition to water. Drinks such as colas, fruit juices, energy drinks and chocolate-flavored beverages often have large amounts of calories and sugar. These unnecessary calories can pack on the pounds. Learn to drink your coffee and tea black or add a small amount of skim milk. Fattening creamers, sweet flavorings, and sugar will add a lot of calories to a naturally calorie-free cup of tea or coffee.

Your Turn

What food will you choose the next time your body signals that it's time to eat between meals? _____

_____

What is your strategy with regard to trigger foods? _____

_____

_____

_____

_____

_____

My Favorite Distraction Techniques

To stop myself from eating when my body didn't need food, I sometimes relaxed in the bathtub or took a hot shower. But I couldn't jump in the tub the eight to ten times a day that hunger struck. When taking a hot bath wasn't convenient, I drank a hot cup of decaffeinated tea or coffee and sucked on a piece of hard candy. Something about the heat and steam of the hot drink relaxed me and helped fill me up. A piece of hard candy has only about 10 calories, and because I made certain not to chew the candy quickly, it lasted a long time and made me happy. If sugar is a concern for you, keep some sugar-free candies at hand.

Whether you choose to eat one portion of a good filling snack, move your body a bit, drink something, or just wait until the urge to eat passes, the most important thing is having a plan. When false hunger strikes, and it will, you can strike back with a positive action plan.

Whether you are physically hungry or desiring to eat from emotional hunger, practice the program of stop, evaluate, and wait that I outlined previously. In repeating this practice, you're developing a new habit. Working your plan will help you avoid making a food mistake that you will immediately regret. It won't be long before you feel that no food is worth the disgust you experience after eating something you know you don't need.

It's your choice how you handle your feelings of hunger. Are you going to give in to emotional hunger and make a choice you will regret, or will you work through your false hunger and come through it feeling good about yourself and the choices you make? Remember my food stash? Even though I was hiding the food, all those calories still counted. Hiding your eating habits doesn't make them go away. Bring them out, turn them over, and put the bad ones aside.

The Importance of Support

When you are learning to make changes in your food choices; practicing the stop, evaluate, and wait principle; and working hard to conquer the emotions that sometimes drive you to overeat, you will likely discover the importance of support. I found enormous support through my husband, my church family, and some of my friends. Although I did not ask them for dieting advice, I did ask them to babysit kids for me on occasion and to not prepare foods I'd be tempted by. I also relied on them to be my cheerleaders as the weight dropped and my success became apparent.

While John was a tremondous help, you may find, as I did, that a good friend can be worth his or her weight in gold. Having someone to talk to about the struggles you are experiencing with certain foods, and knowing that your friend will not judge you if you make a mistake, can be a comfort. I found that when I expressed my feelings verbally, it was a healing experience. John gave me support and made me feel like I was not alone in my journey.

Communication with your support group, whether it is one person or a large number, will remain important as you lose weight. Decide whether you want this group to ask how you are doing on your plan or whether you want to be the initiator of such conversations. If you do not want your friends or family members asking you questions, tell each person what makes you comfortable. I did not want people asking me how I was faring but did want to ask for help if I needed it.

You might want to meet with a counselor to explore some of the emotional struggles you have surrounding food. If you decide to seek counseling, look for a counselor who specializes in weight loss. Do not be afraid to meet with several different counselors until you find a person you feel comfortable with.

12

Habits That Heal,
Habits That Hurt

A re your habits life-bearing? By that I mean: Do your habits improve your life? Do they have a positive impact on your life or on the life of someone else? I don't know about you, but I want to make a difference to the people around me. I want everything I do to have a positive effect on my world. If you're like me and you strive to be a better person, why does it seem impossible to conquer your bad habits when it comes to food?

When I was overweight and obese, my food habits were horrible and unhealthy. Name any bad food habit, and I probably had it at one point or another. Eating after dinner—check. Eating when I wasn't hungry—been there. Frequently overeating—definitely. Substituting food for emotional discomfort—always. Food habits are quick to develop and slow to die. And because food is readily available, and everyone needs food to live, it is easy to develop some bad food habits.

Food consumption and food choices come from ingrained behaviors and emotional needs. The behavioral component often manifests itself in habits such as putting too much food on your plate at dinner or eating large snacks before you go to bed. The emotions that surround food choices can also lead to unhealthy food habits. For example, if you eat candy every time you feel bored, you have likely developed a habit based on emotions.

Established food habits can take a long time to change. According to some research, it takes twenty-one days to drop a habit and forty-two days for a new habit to start becoming part of your routine.

The Euphoria of High-Fat Foods

Some people say that once they start eating high-fat or high-sugar foods, it's hard to stop. It seems that breaking the cycle of unhealthy fat and sugar consumption has some similarities to breaking other types of addictions.

When you consume foods such as ice cream, rich chocolate cake, pound cake, candy bars, or fried apple pie, your brain gets a signal to release endorphins. Endorphins are present in your body naturally and give you a feeling of pleasure. Exercise also signals your brain to release endorphins.

Researchers have found that when you eat large quantities of fats and sugars, your nerve receptors become less receptive to endorphins. Thus you need more sugar and fat to attain the feeling of euphoria you have come to crave.

I found this to be true, both during my years of obesity and during my weight-loss experience. The more chocolate and candy I consumed, the more my body and brain seemed to desire it. Eliminating chocolate from my diet caused strong cravings that I had to resist. Over a period of a few weeks, as my body began to accept the endorphins my brain naturally made, my cravings for chocolate decreased. If you find it hard to resist high-fat, high-sugar foods, know that the desire for those foods will lessen over time.

Your Turn

Are you willing to take the time necessary to break your unhealthy food habits?.. Yes ❑ No ❑

Name at least one habit that you can commit to changing over the next several weeks. _____

_____

_____

_____

You Change Them All the Time

Think about the saying, "You can't teach an old dog new tricks." I know from experience that it is possible to teach new tricks to an old dog, but it is certainly not easy. That's because the longer you have a habit, the more difficult it is to alter. So does that make us old dogs? Kind of. We can teach ourselves some new tricks when it comes to food. It just takes some time and effort.

People change their habits all the time—but not always deliberately. Often, life events force us to develop new habits. If you have children, think back to when they were born. In my case, almost every routine I had developed prior to having children had to change afterward. My sleeping habits changed, my lengthy showers shortened, my social activities changed—all because of a tiny bundle who needed me. I changed my long-established habits willingly and enthusiastically because I loved that baby more than life itself. In addition, I realized that my day-to-day routines would be easier with new habits designed to accommodate her. If we can change for another person, why is it so hard to change for ourselves?

Have you ever moved from one house or apartment to another? Remember when you were deciding where to store the plates, cups, and bowls? Can you remember how long it took before you stopped opening random cabinets, trying to find the coffee mugs? I'd wager it took a good six weeks (forty-two days) before you got the new routine down pat. We have moved numerous times, and each time that's about how long it took me to consistently remember where things were.

Food Habits

You are working on changing your food habits, and that's going to take some time. When I was losing weight, it took at least six weeks to make the new food choices part of my daily routine. Once you realign your thinking and change your habits, you begin to feel confident that you can win at weight loss. Eating is an emotional experience for many people, and emotional habits can be difficult to break and keep broken. Food habits are near and dear to us, familiar and safe. Although changing long-established habits is challenging, you can do it, one by one.

Your Turn

Make a list of your current food habits, such as eating at certain times of the day, reaching for the same foods over and over, eating sweets after dinner, or always ordering the same entrée at a restaurant:_____

_____

_____

_____

Commit to replacing your food habits with healthy food habits. For example, if you always have a sweet dessert after dinner, replace it with fresh fruit. List your replacement habits here:_____

_____

_____

Confession Brownies

When I was fat, chocolate was a friend who never failed me. If I had a bad day, I would reach for the chocolate. If I had a good day—let's celebrate with chocolate! Chocolate was a habit for me, and I ate it at all times of day, often without thinking about what I was doing. That's the very definition of a habit, isn't it? A recurrent, often unconscious pattern of behavior acquired through frequent repetition. Well, I certainly frequently repeated that pattern.

I'd like to share a little story to illustrate how much I loved chocolate. Years ago, I would not only plan dinner for the evening, I would also plan dessert. Sometimes I'd make a pan of brownies early in the day, with the intention of serving them for dessert that night. But many times the brownies didn't last past lunchtime. Over the course of several hours, I'd have a corner here and a bite there. Before I knew it, an entire row of brownies was gone. Well, then I needed to go ahead and get rid of the rest of them, so that John wouldn't know I had eaten a whole row. Before I knew it, the whole pan was gone. I would then race around like a mad woman, trying to bake another pan before John came home, so he wouldn't know I had eaten an entire pan of brownies by myself. On those occasions, he would often remark how nice it was to have the dessert warm.

What we came to call confession brownies came about by accident. Once I was making brownies late in the day. This time, I added chocolate frosting. The pan looked beautiful, with the smooth shiny chocolate frosting glistening as it dried. Although I tried to resist, I began my usual picking at the corners. Without even realizing it, I had eaten about half a row. On this day I had a problem, because I didn't have enough time to make an additional pan. And the beautiful smooth shiny frosting was now a globby mess, as I unsuccessfully tried to resmooth it into the gap where the missing brownies had been. The more I moved the frosting around, the worse it looked. Slam! The door opened and closed and John was home. Yikes.

He said, "Is that brownies I smell?"

I nodded. He was excited, as were the children. We sat down to eat dinner. The whole time I was sitting there, I wondered how I could avoid confessing what I had done. When everyone had eaten dinner, I got up to cut the brownies. As I stood at the kitchen counter looking at the globby frosting, I realized you can't cover up mistakes. So I bravely walked back to the table and plopped the whole pan down. I told the family, "I have a confession to make." I explained what I had done and how I had tried to cover up my mistake by moving the frosting around, but it hadn't worked. We all had a good laugh about it and coined the name "confession brownies" for brownies with frosting.

When I make confession brownies now, anyone who wants to can confess something without any repercussions. The kids are usually funny and tell stories about themselves and each other. Eating confession brownies has become a fun, family time, and we all end up laughing and talking at once.

The lesson I learned from confession brownies is this: You may think, as I did, that no one sees your bad habits. And they might not. But *you* see what mistakes you make with your food choices, and the repercussions are both external and internal. The external consequences make themselves widely known as your weight slowly creeps up. In some ways, the internal consequences are even worse, as you feel guilty for making bad choices and breaking promises to yourself (which in turn might make you unhappy and make you want to eat).

Strange Habits

As I was finally getting on track with my weight loss, I discovered a funny habit I didn't even know I had. I realized that every time I answered the phone, I automatically headed to the pantry and opened the door. I would stand there, talking on the phone, looking into the pantry. If the phone call lasted more than a few minutes, I looked into boxes, trying to find something to eat. My poor friends and family on the other end of the phone heard me chewing or crunching for the rest of the conversation. Hopefully you don't have this habit, because, according to my husband, it's very rude. I always tried to chew quietly, but I guess I wasn't fooling anyone. After all, potato chips are hard to eat silently.

As you go about your daily routine over the next few weeks, look for those unexpected and unexplainable habits. My eating-on-the-phone habit took me by surprise, and it was difficult to break. Even to this day, I often find myself standing in the walk-in pantry when I'm on the phone. Then I shake my head, leave the pantry, and close the door, thinking, *What am I doing in here?* The next time you find yourself eating due to a strange food habit, think, *What am I doing here?*

Habits of Deception

In my Fit to the Finish program, many participants share that they deceived people about the quantity or types of food they were eating. When I was overweight, I often felt like people were watching every morsel of food I put in my mouth, from the first bite to the last. I was probably imagining it, but that's how I felt. Consequently, when dining with friends, I was very careful about the amount of food I put on my plate. After all, I was always on some type of diet, and I wanted people to think I was in control of my food intake—right? Secondly, I didn't want them to think I was a pig. Thirdly, I thought if people didn't see me eat very much, perhaps they would assume I was fat because I had some type of metabolism problem or a thyroid issue. When we left the dinner party or friends left our house, I was always famished. I was accustomed to eating a lot more food than I had just consumed. Once John and I got home or the company had left, I would head directly to the kitchen and begin foraging.

I wonder now what John thought as I opened the pantry and began to eat again. In only a few minutes, I would have chips, ice cream, and cookies. I remember heating up hot fudge sauce to pour over full-fat ice cream at eleven at night after a dinner out. Eating the sticky hot fudge gave me comfort, but I went to bed with an overly full stomach and a guilty conscience.

Your Turn

Have you ever eaten a meal with friends or family and eaten less than you would have had you been alone?..Yes ❑ No ❑

If so, why did you do this? _____
_____
_____

How did it make you feel? _____
_____
_____

Did you eat again later?.. Yes ❑ No ❑

If yes, what did you eat and how much? _____
_____
_____

Car Habits

If you're eating in your car, more likely than not, you're eating unhealthy foods. Fast food, convenience store foods, and takeout foods are usually high in fat, contain an astronomical amount of calories, and have enough sodium to fulfill your requirement for a week.

For many people, eating while driving is a matter of convenience. It is undoubtedly easier to grab a value meal while you are running errands than it is to pack a snack. It's fun, in the short term, to stock up on a little treat while pumping gas. But those seemingly easy choices can be detrimental to long-term goals and objectives.

I knew my habit of eating in the car wasn't the best choice for me, but I couldn't seem to stop. After all, I had had a decade to develop this bad habit. In fact, the habit was so important to me that I often ate food in the car that I wouldn't dream of eating in front of John. Even though John and I ate together in the evenings, he had no idea that I often ate two lunches and two dinners when he was at work. When I weighed about 260 pounds, I remember inventing an excuse to run an errand, just so I could go to Wendy's and order a large Frosty and some fries. I was so engrossed in eating while driving back home that I almost forgot to get the item I had supposedly gone on the errand to get. I remember thinking that I didn't even taste the food because I ate it so quickly to avoid getting caught.

When I started my plan, I couldn't simply say, "I'm never going to eat in the car again, unless we are on a trip." Merely saying those words wouldn't magically erase a habit I had taken years to perfect. Instead, I developed an alternative plan of attack. I used the same stop, evaluate, and wait pattern for fast food that I used for determining whether I was feeling physical or emotional hunger.

When I was driving and the desire for fast food struck, I would ask myself if I was really hungry or if I just wanted fries, a shake, or a sandwich. Usually, I wasn't actually hungry, as I had recently eaten a meal. In the past, that wouldn't have stopped me, but this time I had a strong desire to change. I was training myself in a new way of thinking. After admitting that I wasn't really hungry, I would force myself to continue driving past the restaurant that had triggered my desire for fast food. By the time the next row of fast-food restaurants came into view, I had given myself a little talk about whether or not I was really hungry and about making a better choice. Usually, believe it or not, the plan worked. Each time I said no, my confidence became more emboldened. I felt a little more in control and less of a slave to my appetite. With practice, I replaced a bad habit with the good one of continuing down the road without pulling into the drive-through lane of a restaurant.

My tactic worked because I didn't automatically tell myself no. Instead, I told myself to wait and gave myself time to think about what I was really hungry for. If I was truly hungry, I could almost always wait a few more minutes, until I could get home and have a healthy snack. The tactic didn't always work, but nine times out of ten, I resisted the urge to eat junk. The times I did pull into the drive-through lane, I felt so guilty that I'd give most of the food to the kids and eat only a few fries. Over time, it became easier and easier to resist temptation and break that bad habit.

Your Turn

Do you ever eat in the car? .... Yes ❏ No ❏

If so, what do you eat? _____

_____

_____

Is this the best choice? .... Yes ❏ No ❏

Is there a fast-food restaurant you find hard to resist? .... Yes ❏ No ❏
What can you do to avoid drive-through dangers? _____

_____

_____

Grocery Shopping Habits

Kids are smart, and although they say they can't hear us when we call them from the next room, they can hear a candy wrapper being opened 25 feet away. My older children in particular realized that Mommy ate too much. Whenever I bought chips, candy, or cookies at the grocery store, my oldest daughter would ask, "Mommy, are you going to eat all those chips, or will I get some too?" I would always laugh and tell her she was so silly, but she was right. It was my habit to go grocery shopping, buy lots of delicious snacks and candies, and then, before the car left the parking lot, start munching away on whatever box my hand touched first. Sometimes I even kept track of the big yellow bag of Peanut M&M's as it passed down the checkout conveyor belt to see which sack the clerk put it in, so I could easily find the candy and eat it on the way home. It was just another habit that I developed over the years, and one that was quite hard to break.

To break the habit of purchasing candy, I started avoiding certain aisles in the grocery store. The healthier food choices tend to be on the outer perimeter of the store. In many grocery stores, the produce, dairy products, meats, nuts and seeds, and breads are located along the outer perimeter, while the inner aisles mostly contain processed foods with fat, sugar, and preservatives. By not traveling down the cookie or chip aisle, I avoided the temptation to throw a box or two in the cart. The kids benefited by having healthier snacks, and I benefited by not having to see the tempting food—assuming I could resist the end caps, with their artful displays of cookies, sugary cereals, and fattening crackers. I wrote down my complete grocery store list before I left the house and stuck to it. For the kids I bought treats that I wasn't very fond of and that I could easily say no to. While shopping, I rarely added any extra food to my cart. Over time, I became a health-conscious shopper and a wise consumer. I learned what was healthy and what wasn't, and my entire family benefited.

As the primary shopper in my family, I realized that I had almost complete control over what foods ended up in my shopping cart. This was a humbling realization for me, as I had to acknowledge that all 99 percent of the junk that had previously been living in my pantry and refrigerator was there because of me. If you are the primary shopper, take advantage of your role by making the best choices you can. If someone else shops alongside you, or for you, make an effort to clearly communicate what types of foods are desirable and give him or her tips on making healthy choices by shopping the perimeter of the store and reading food labels.

Your Turn

Do you buy particular foods for yourself at the
grocery store?.. Yes ❑ No ❑

Are these the best choices for you?.. Yes ❑ No ❑

If you answered "no," what can you do to stop the temptation to purchase these particular foods? _____

_____

_____

Do you shop mostly the inner aisles of the grocery
store or the outer aisles?...Inner ❏ Outer ❏

If you selected the inner aisles, can you make a grocery list that includes
mainly whole foods located on the outer perimeter of the store? _____

_____

_____

_____

_____

If you are the primary shopper in your family, is it feasible to have someone else do the grocery shopping for the household? .... Yes ❏ No ❏

The Eating-after-Dinner Habit

Once I started to lose weight the last time, my best line of defense against
late-night snacking was to keep busy long enough for the urge to pass. I
didn't stop watching television but was mindful to ignore commercials
that featured my favorite foods. I distracted myself by brushing and floss-
ing my teeth, drinking a cup of hot tea, scrapbooking, knitting, or talking
to family on the phone. The majority of the time, I would win the war on
eating after dinner. Breaking this habit was extremely beneficial to me,
as it limited the number of calories I consumed, helped me sleep more
soundly, and gave me one less thing to feel guilty about.

Even now, more than a decade after I lost my weight, I rarely eat after
dinner. If I want dessert, I have it while the family is sitting at the table. If
I don't eat it then, I don't eat it at all.

Your Turn

Do you eat after dinner? .... Yes ❏ No ❏

What do you eat? _____

_____

_____

How many times a week? _____

_____

What strategy will you employ to avoid eating after your evening meal?

_____

_____

What benefits will you see as a result of breaking this habit? _____

_____

_____

Is there someone you can ask to help you stay honest and
consistent with your food habits?.. Yes ❏ No ❏

Establishing New Habits

Staying in the weight-loss game requires some creative thinking. One time when I had just begun my weight-loss journey, I "accidentally" bought some cookies I liked. I gave the unopened package to the children and asked them to hide the cookies in a secret place and no matter what, not to tell me where they were. Imagine my annoyance when one hour later, I asked the kids where the cookies were and they wouldn't tell me. I hid my annoyance and said, "I was just checking to see if you were still playing the game!" Those children could really hide things—darn.

Although I could enlist the help of John and the children, and they were often very helpful, I couldn't rely on them to police my eating habits. I needed to work on each and every bad habit as it revealed itself. I needed to take that habit "out of the closet," look at it long and hard, and decide on a plan of action to get rid of it.

You know what? It worked, and I haven't gone back to any of those old habits. It wasn't overnight that I quit eating when I was bored, stressed, or on the phone. It took a good six weeks to see a change in how I responded to those situations. It took constant work and constant reassessment of each situation. I couldn't just tell myself I wasn't going to eat in the car

Dealing with Unsupportive or Sabotaging Partners

I was lucky that I had a supportive partner when I was losing weight. While John did eat junk with me when I was obese, once I started losing weight, he rarely complained about the lack of junky snacks in the house or asked me to purchase candy or ice cream. But John did feel some insecurities as I went from a size 26/28 to a size 6/8. He worried that I would not want to stay with him after I was slim and fit—an unfounded concern.

You may not be as lucky as I was. You might have a partner who brings you candy as a treat after a hard day, goads you into eating more food than you planned to eat in a restaurant, or teases you when you refuse to eat what he or she is eating. One woman's husband told his friends how proud he was of his wife for trying to lose weight, but at the same time he brought her pints of gourmet ice cream, asked her to fry chicken rather than bake it, and served her extremely large portions of food at dinner. He was clearly experiencing insecurity with his wife's changing lifestyle and appearance and wanted things to stay how they had always been. Their marriage did not last.

Communicating with your spouse about your expectations is the first step in dealing with these problems. Explain that you do not want him or her to unintentionally sabotage your weight loss efforts by bringing home candy or chips. Ask your partner how he or she feels about the changes you are making. Discuss together how your partner can support you without bringing you food.

Involve your spouse in your journey, even if he or she does not need to lose weight. Work in the kitchen together, preparing lower-calorie, lower-fat versions of your favorite foods. Ask your partner to take walks or bike rides with you.

If your spouse seems intent on outwardly ridiculing you or steadily sabotaging your efforts, consider seeking the counsel of a pastor or a psychologist who can help you both deal with your changing appearance and lifestyle.

anymore and declare the problem solved. I had to have an actual plan of what to do when faced with the temptation to give in to one of my bad eating habits.

You can do it too. Review your answers to the questions in this chapter and then answer the following:

Your Turn

Which of your food habits bothers you the most? _____
_____
_____
_____

Why do you think this one bothers you more than other ones? _____
_____
_____
_____

What are three ideas you have to change that habit this week? _____
_____
_____
_____

Work on one habit at a time, and you will be surprised how quickly you are ready to tackle the next one. It is stressful to change everything in your life at once, but by steadily working through one bad habit at a time, you will make progress. And once you see progress, you will build the momentum and motivation for more positive changes.

Final Thoughts

You can improve and change your habits because you are always changing things in your life. Think of your food habits as ones you just haven't achieved a high level of control over yet. You can take control of your bad habits and change them for the better. It's important to give yourself a mental pat on the back when you make progress in conquering a bad habit. Only you can change your habits. No one else can do it for you.

If I can give you just one piece of encouragement, it would be this: A habit is just that—a habit. It's only a way of doing something. Just because you do something now doesn't mean you have to be controlled by that behavior forever. You can change for the better. Wouldn't you rather it be by choice than by force? Wouldn't you rather hear your doctor say, "Good job" than, "If you don't get your blood pressure under control with diet and exercise, we are going to have to put you on medication?" Make the choice to change for you. One day at a time.

13

Waiting on a Plateau

As you continue on your journey toward fitness, your weight loss might come to a screeching halt. If this happens, you have hit the dreaded plateau—a period when your weight loss stops. Your plateau might last a week or a month. Sometimes I think the real person's definition of a plateau should be: "A time all people trying to lose weight dread." Plateauing is one of the most frustrating experiences you can have while losing weight, as there is something inherently difficult about continuing a plan when the plan does not seem to be working.

Plateauing is frustrating, but it is normal. Almost every person who loses weight eventually reaches a plateau. Why? In the initial weight-loss phase, you often lose weight quickly as your body releases extra water weight. After the initial period of "easy" weight loss, your body begins burning fat and some muscle tissue. This process often slows down your weight loss to a reasonable .5 to 2 pounds a week. Over time, however, your metabolism begins to slow down as you lose muscle and you reach the balance point between caloric intake and weight maintenance. Once you reach this point, your weight loss stalls.

The weight-loss process is a physical process, but staying committed to your weight loss in the face of a plateau involves engaging your emotional side as well. To conquer a plateau, you need to focus on your goals, on getting the scale to move again, and on being honest with yourself.

Your Turn

Do you weigh yourself every day (or every week)? .... Yes ❑ No ❑

Do you own a good, accurate scale? .... Yes ❑ No ❑

How do you feel when you step on a scale and see that you have lost a few pounds? _____

_____

After such a weight loss, do you expect to continue losing weight at the same rate? .... Yes ❑ No ❑

Why or why not? _____

_____

Has your weight plateaued during a time when you were trying to lose weight? .... Yes ❑ No ❑

How did you feel when your weight loss stopped after you were having some measure of success? _____

_____

What action did you take when you realized your weight-loss progress had slowed or stopped? _____

_____

Why did you react the way you did? _____

_____

Could you have reacted in a way that would have been more effective? .... Yes ❑ No ❑

Did you continue in your quest to lose weight? .... Yes ❑ No ❑

Why or why not? _____

_____

Dealing with Plateaus

Plateaus occur whether you have 150 pounds to lose, as I did, or whether you have 10 pounds to lose. Plateaus are inevitable. And if you think about it, they make sense. We don't gain the 10, 20, or 30 pounds overnight, or with perfect consistency, so why should we expect to lose those same 10, 20, or 30 pounds without some stalling along the way?

It can be depressing to finally lose some weight and then hit a plateau. At that point, you might even give up on your weight-loss plan and quickly gain back all the weight you lost, plus a few bonus pounds. When I was first dieting, I tried to convince myself that my weight had hit a plateau because that was the weight where my body was happy. I reasoned that trying to lose weight beyond that number was futile. I deceived myself by not looking honestly at my lifestyle and eating habits. I gave up. Don't you give up. It is almost always possible to push past a plateau and have long-term success. To avoid the dieting cycle, you must plan how you will react when your weight loss stalls.

After many weight-loss plateaus, I realized that I hated plateaus in all areas of my life. When I was single and dating, I hated the times of "coasting" in a relationship. I either wanted the relationship to move along or end. I also got frustrated when my career seemed to stall. Then I would start toying with the idea of looking for another job. I disliked it when I worked on a new skill, such as playing the piano, and my level of expertise stalled. I had to make the choice to either practice more or give up. I realized that it was not just weight-loss plateaus that frustrated me. I did not like being stalled in any area of life.

With this newfound understanding, I began my diet the final time, accepting that I would hit plateaus and that that would be okay. I realized if I were going to be successful, I needed to exert both willpower and self-discipline: willpower to resist eating when I should not and self-discipline to continue on my journey in the face of little progress. Changing my lifestyle and radically altering my eating habits proved to be both simple and difficult.

It was simple to decide what things I wanted to change. I knew I was eating too much unhealthy fat, too many calories, and not enough healthy foods. I understood the problem. The hard part was following through with my program pound after pound, day after day, month after month.

But I found that success breeds success. You will likely find that once you have endured and passed one plateau, the next will be slightly easier to handle. The feelings of discouragement and the temptation to give up will be replaced by the knowledge that you can continue on your weight-loss journey without quitting.

Your Turn

How does the following statement make you feel? *I accept the fact that plateaus are part of weight loss.* _____

_____

_____

_____

_____

Are you willing to persevere in your weight-loss plan despite
the inevitable plateaus? .... Yes ❑ No ❑

Do you agree or disagree with this statement: *Weight loss
is a combination of willpower and self-discipline* ....Agree ❑ Disagree ❑

Do you have the tools to be successful for the long haul? .... Yes ❑ No ❑

When No One Notices

I began my diet in 1997 by cutting out unhealthy foods and committing to daily exercise. Because I was so heavy, the weight came off quickly in the beginning. I had some early success, which helped me stay motivated. The frustrating part was that no one, not even me, could tell I had lost any weight. After losing 20 pounds, I still wore the same big pants, still looked fat, and still had not received a single compliment. At the 40-pound mark, even John was unaware I had lost any weight. I stood on the scale one morning soon after losing 40 pounds and realized that I had not lost any weight in four or five days. I could not believe it. I had been following my plan! I had not missed a single day of exercise, and I had not eaten anything too terrible.

In the past, I would have used this plateau as another excuse to quit. This time, because I had mentally prepared myself for the inevitable hills, valleys, and plateaus, I kept going. Instead of giving up when the scale stalled, I kept following my plan. To my surprise, the weight loss continued. Finally, after the weight loss plateau ended and I had lost about 10 more pounds, two people noticed. They tentatively asked, "Have you lost some weight?" Talk about motivating! Now I was on fire, ready to push past any other plateaus and get my excess weight off. I stayed focused and did all the right things, but eventually the weight loss stopped again. What had I done wrong? Nothing. I was in the wait part of weight loss. If you stick with any diet for a period of time, you too will experience a plateau. The timing is different for each person.

It was not easy to look at the same number on the scale for days. I could have been depressed, mad, or frustrated. In the past, I would have been all of those things and more. I would have gone straight to the pantry, flung open the door, and said, "Well, if I'm going to do all this work and not lose any weight, I might as well eat anything I want." But this time I didn't. I thought about what I had learned over the previous few months. I remembered that I had experienced plateaus in many areas of life throughout the years and did not always give up. I knew I wanted to lose weight more than anything. So I resisted the call of the pantry. Was I proud? You bet I was. Every other time I had dieted long enough to hit a plateau, my first reaction was to eat. This time I achieved a major victory by resisting and not running to food for comfort.

That first plateau lasted ten long days. But as quickly as it started, it was over, and I began seeing the scale go down again.

Your Turn

Do you have a plan for handling plateaus during your
dieting attempts? .... Yes ❑ No ❑

What have you done in the past when your weight loss stopped? _____
_____

Did it work? .... Yes ❑ No ❑

What Got Me Here

Planning is very important during all stages of weight loss. It's important to plan meals, have strategies for handling holidays, and have a plan for those inevitable plateaus. Without a comprehensive plan, your weight-loss attempt will fail. What should you do when your weight loss comes to a screeching halt? In this chapter, I share some strategies to help you conquer the plateaus to come.

First things first: Get out of the kitchen! I normally headed right for the pantry when things got tough. After I decided to leave the kitchen, I had another choice to make. I could choose to overeat and undo the good work I had started, or I could choose *not* to run to food.

When you are tempted to run to food in the face of a plateau, force yourself to go anywhere but the kitchen. Now that you are out of the kitchen, think logically, read the suggestions that follow, and make some decisions. First, ask yourself these four questions:

Have You Followed Your Eating Plan?

Have you eaten more than 30 percent of your calories from fat? Have you binged? Could you be falling into a common fat trap: eating too much low-fat food, forgetting that low fat does not equal low calories?

If you keep a food diary, examine it closely to see if overeating could be the reason you have stopped losing weight. If you don't keep a food diary, take a few minutes to honestly think about what you have been eating. Use the food diary in appendix F. Sometimes, just by writing down your recent food choices, you can readily see where the problem lies.

By the way, it doesn't do any good to be dishonest with yourself. You can try convincing yourself the half package of Double Stuff Oreos you ate two days ago didn't affect your weight loss, but you are only hurting yourself. Take ownership of your food choices, both bad and good. If you realize you have been eating too many high-fat foods, resolve to stop. If a particular food, such as chocolate, is tripping you up, rid your house of that food. I know it's wasteful, but just throw it in the trash and drop a raw egg on top of it, so you won't be tempted to retrieve it from the can and eat it. If the foods you have been overindulging in are low-fat choices but you've just been eating too much of them, go back to measuring your food for a week. Visually remind yourself that one portion of pasta shouldn't look like a little mountain sitting on your plate.

Have You Been Exercising?

This is an easy one. Either yes, you've been exercising, or no, you've stopped. As you know, exercise burns calories. As long as you are not replacing those calories with food, a good exercise program will help you lose weight—not only through burning calories but also through building muscle (which helps your body burn calories more efficiently).

If you haven't begun exercising and your weight loss has hit a plateau, check with your doctor. If he or she gives you the green light to exercise, then start. Exercise is one of the most important parts of a weight-loss plan. You will find it to be more and more pleasurable as time goes on. Even if you abhor exercise when you start, keep with it for at least six weeks. You might even start looking forward to your exercise sessions.

If you have been exercising and your weight loss has hit a plateau, you might need to step up your exercise. Your body is getting smaller and accustomed to a certain level of movement. The result is that it uses fewer calories and expends less energy. Just as a smaller car uses less fuel, a person who weighs less requires fewer calories than a person who weighs more. That alone could be the reason for the plateau. So it's important, with your doctor's okay, to step up your level of exercise as it gets easier. Start exercising more vigorously and vary your exercise routine to get your weight loss going again.

Is There Another Explanation?

Can you think of any other reason your weight loss has stalled? For example, I found it difficult to lose weight during the week prior to my menstrual cycle. As I mentioned earlier, in the week leading up to menstruation, some chemical reactions in the brain tell the body that it's hungry. If you are a man, you can't use this excuse.

Another possible reason for the plateau could be too many diet drinks. I could always tell when I drank too many diet drinks because my fingers swelled slightly and I felt a little puffy. You know that feeling—almost like there is an extra layer of fluid under your skin. I don't drink many diet drinks these days, but during my weight-loss year, I sometimes drank too much Diet Coke. If you have been drinking a lot of carbonated beverages, try cutting back and increasing your water intake. You should be drinking at least six to eight glasses of water per day. An added benefit to drinking lots of water is that if you are properly hydrated, you tend to eat less.

Stress can also stall weight loss. When you are stressed, your body secretes a hormone called cortisol. Cortisol can increase appetite, making it difficult to control your caloric intake. In addition, research suggests that high cortisol levels may result in increased abdominal fat. Stress can affect your eating habits. If you think stress is affecting your weight loss, try some stress-reduction techniques such as deep breathing, a hot bath, a weekly massage, or having a conversation you've been putting off.

Have You Been Eating Enough Food?

Metabolism changes as your weight changes, and if you consistently eat too little, your body will rebel. Remember, losing weight is purely a matter of math: you must burn more calories than you consume. So you might think the less you eat, the faster you will lose weight, right? That logic goes only so far, because your metabolism isn't static—it adjusts to your activity level, how much you eat, your percentage of muscle mass, certain hormones, and other factors. Your body's goal is to maintain its current weight. When you start cutting down on what you eat, your metabolism adjusts by slowing down, so you don't burn as many calories as you had been burning.

If you cut your calorie consumption too drastically, you will lose some weight, but after a while you won't be losing the right type of weight. You will be losing muscle. You want to lose fat, not muscle, and moderation is the key. A safe level of calorie reduction is to cut 100 to 200 calories from your daily intake, making certain that you consume at least 1,200 calories. This reduction will often be enough to get your weight loss started again.

Make sure the food you do eat is nutritious, including lots of lean protein, vegetables, and fruit. Cut way back on refined sugar and simple starches, foods that are highly processed, and sugar-filled desserts. A moderate amount of fat—up to 30 percent of your daily calories—is appropriate, as long as only 7 percent of it is saturated fat.

At the same time, increase the amount of calories you're burning by 200 to 300 per day. Do a half hour to an hour of moderate exercise, such as brisk walking, jogging, dancing, or swimming. Remember that the more intense the activity, the less time you need to spend at it. Make sure you include some resistance training, or strength training, to keep up your muscle mass and help your metabolism stay elevated throughout the day.

As a rule of thumb, women should not go below 1,200 calories per day for weight loss, and men should not go below 1,500. But what if you've messed up, and you're on that unhealthy 800- to 1,000-calorie diet? Don't worry, you can fix it. Remember, metabolism isn't static. It fluctuates in either direction. Gradually start adding more calories to your diet, maybe 50 to 100 at a time. Since your metabolism has slowed, if you immediately go back to a normal diet, your starving body will cling to every calorie and you will put on weight. So slowly add the calories back to reach a healthy level. Stay only lightly active, because when your calorie intake is too low, you should not exercise intensely. Interestingly, people sometimes find they start losing weight again when they begin adding calories back— because their bodies are no longer in starvation mode.

When you are back to eating a reasonable amount of calories (1,500 to 1,600 for most women who want to lose weight; 1,800 to 2,000 calories for most men), you can start adjusting your activity level and caloric intake.

Your Turn

Have you hit weight-loss plateaus in the past? .... Yes ❑ No ❑
What can you do differently this time? _____
_____
_____

As a reminder, rewrite the four questions to ask yourself when you hit a plateau: _____
_____
_____
_____

Once I asked myself the four questions, and honestly answered each one, I could usually see the reason for my plateau. If you see the probable cause, take steps immediately to resolve the issue. Don't wait until tomorrow to throw bad food away, exercise more, eat less, or monitor your calorie intake. Start today and you will soon see progress.

Patience Required

What happens if you hit a plateau, ask the right questions, and take action, but the scale still doesn't move in the right direction? Remind yourself that weight loss is a journey and that one or two days of healthy eating and exercise can't erase two weeks of overindulgence. Patience is important while you work on modifying your weight-loss plan.

Take stock of how far you've come. You need to be your own cheerleader, because no one else knows exactly what you looked like before you started changing your lifestyle, and no one knows all the little victories you've experienced along the way. No one but me knew all the times I resisted the little temptations that came my way while I was losing weight.

Focus on Nonscale Victoria

I remember once when Rachel went to a birthday party and came home with a "goody bag." She eagerly dumped the contents on the kitchen counter and proudly counted all the little pieces of candy. I looked on with mild interest, until the Hershey's Kisses came tumbling out. Oh dear, I loved those, and she knew it. She looked up at me with those big brown eyes and said, "Mommy, do you want one of these?" It took everything I had not to snatch that silver Kiss out of her little hand. I calmly said, "No, sweetie, Mommy doesn't want one." That was a victory for me. When I hit plateaus, I looked back on that victory and reminded

Six Tips for Conquering Plateaus

Once you've fixed the obvious problems, here are some more tips to get your weight loss going once again.

1. Mix Up Your Calorie Intake

Try changing your day-to-day calorie intake while maintaining the same weekly intake. Let's say you usually eat about 1,600 calories a day. Try eating 1,400 one day, 1,600 the next, and 1,800 the third day. That simple step can sometimes help break a plateau.

2. Start Lifting Weights

Working your muscles will help strengthen bone tissue, increase lean muscle mass, and ultimately boost your metabolic rate. Muscle burns calories faster than fat does.

3. Change It Up

Walking is a great exercise, but your body can get accustomed to a certain amount of activity and effort. Try confusing your body by jogging, swimming, or cycling. The activity doesn't matter, as long as you are doing something strenuous and new.

4. Alter Macronutrient Intake

Macronutrients include proteins, fats, and carbohydrates. Your body needs these important nutrients in larger amounts than micronutrients such as iron, vitamin C, and folate. Slightly change the balance of carbohydrates, proteins, and fats that you eat each day. If your diet consists mostly of carbohydrates, try eating fewer carbs and more protein. If you change it up a bit, your body may respond positively. Don't increase or decrease calories significantly, just the types of food you are eating.

5. Change Your Meals

If you always eat three meals a day, at the same time every day, try adding snacks in between (which may mean reducing the portion size of the main meals). Eating more often is an excellent way to increase your metabolism.

6. Think about Something Else

Relax and take the pressure off. It is easy to focus too much on the number on the scale. I found that if I focused on something other than my weight, the weight eventually started to come off again.

myself that I didn't want to waste my hard work by eating something I knew I'd regret.

At this point, take your measurements again. Put on an outfit that has gotten looser. I can't tell you how many times I tried on my wedding dress during those months of weight loss. At first I couldn't even get it over my shoulders. Then I could get it on but couldn't zip the first inch. Eventually, though, the zipper began to meet for longer stretches. By our eleventh anniversary, I could actually put the dress on, zip it up, and walk into the living room. It was a wonderful experience

Focus also on victories attained in the area of physical fitness. If you've begun exercising or stepping up your exercise, what can you do now that you couldn't do at the beginning of your journey? When I first started exercising, it was only for ten minutes at a time. I would huff and puff back up to the house. That was a victory. Once my weight started to come down and my fitness level increased, I could walk at a quick pace for an hour without being exhausted.

Share Yourself

Another helpful technique when dealing with a plateau is to take the focus off yourself and turn your emotional energy to someone else. When I was losing weight, I became somewhat obsessed with myself—with my weight, my clothes, my eating, and my exercise. That's not healthy, either physically or emotionally. So when the scale stopped moving, I'd remind myself that life wasn't all about me. There was always a friend or family member who needed attention or help working through a crisis. When I put my relationship with God and other people first, I found it much easier to put my weight in perspective.

Like everything in life, a plateau during weight loss is a temporary state of affairs. A plateau will eventually pass. In the course of life, a few days or weeks of no weight loss is a minor thing. It is something that is easily corrected. If you let a plateau overwhelm you, you have let the plateau win. You are stronger than that. Remind yourself of how far you've come, not how much further you have to go.

Your Turn

Describe a victory you have experienced during a period of weight loss:

_____

_____

Does anyone else know about it?... Yes ❑ No ❑

How do your measurements now compare to those you recorded when you first started trying to lose weight? _____

_____

_____

Is there an outfit that fits you better now than it did a
few weeks ago? .... Yes ❑ No ❑

What can you do now that you would have found difficult in the past? Think about things such as saying no to certain foods, exercising regularly, or being able to walk farther or more easily. _____

_____

_____

How does that make you feel? _____

_____

_____

Do you know someone who needs your help with meals,
transportation, or a listening ear? .... Yes ❑ No ❑

What is one specific thing you will do this week for someone else?

_____

_____

14

Eating Out without Blowing Up

Furniture designers calculate the size of restaurant booths based on the average size of diners. I, however, was not an average-size diner. The first time I got stuck trying to slide into a restaurant booth was a mortifying experience. A friend and I went shopping one evening and left the children with our respective husbands. We picked a casual cafeteria-style restaurant, one that neither of us had tried before. We walked through the line, made our selections, and paid for our food. The cashier gave us an order number and told us to sit wherever we liked. The server would bring our orders in a few minutes.

We looked around the restaurant and saw booths along the walls and some tables in the middle. My friend pointed out an empty booth and said, "How about that one?"

I said, "Sure." It didn't even cross my mind that an embarrassing situation might be looming in my near future. We walked across the crowded restaurant, put our trays on the table, and decided to get our drinks before sitting down. Walking back across the restaurant to the drink station was uneventful, except that my hips occasionally brushed people's shoulders as I squeezed through the closely packed tables. Once over that hurdle, I arrived back at the table to find my friend already sitting down. I put my drink on the table, bent my knees, leaned down a bit, and started to slide into the booth.

Whoops. There wasn't enough room between the seat and the table for me. My first attempt left me hanging halfway off the seat, with half my bottom on the seat and half in the air. I sucked in my breath and tried to force my way in. It was impossible. My friend looked on in horror as I continued to move around in a vain attempt to fit. I finally settled for hanging my legs over the outside of the booth and kind of sitting on the seat. This was clearly not going to work. At this point, I had attracted some attention—none of which was favorable. My poor friend didn't know what to do. To make matters worse, who should come strolling up but our friendly server, ready to put our meals on the table. She stopped in her tracks when she saw me sitting sideways in the booth. I said, "I think we are going to sit at that table over there rather than in this booth."

She nodded and put our food on the more accommodating table. I scooped up my drink, silverware, purse, and pride and waddled over to the table. My friend was right behind me. What a good friend, to stick with me, even in such an embarrassing situation. Once we were settled at the table, I apologized to her for the embarrassing moment. She just shrugged it off, but the evening was ruined. All I could think about was how stupid I must have looked trying to shove myself into the booth. I could just imagine the stories the other diners would tell their families when they got home. I tried to look on the bright side and appreciate the fact that at least I hadn't recognized anyone in the restaurant. When I got home, I drowned my sorrows in a half gallon of ice cream.

After that experience, I practiced judging the opening between the seat and the table of restaurant booths. I realized that some tables were anchored to the floor, while some could be moved a bit. The ones anchored down were taboo. The moveable tables were okay, as long as I was with a thin friend who could still fit in her seat if I pushed the table toward her. It took years before I finally could sit in a restaurant booth without worrying, *Will I fit?*

Restaurant Calories

When I was growing up, my family did not go to restaurants very often. My mother and father grew up right after the Depression, and they were inclined to save money. So when we did go out to eat, it was a huge treat and was usually for lunch, as evening restaurant meals were reserved for their date nights.

Restaurant foods tend to be richer, higher in fat, and laden with more calories than home-cooked meals. If you eat at a restaurant only a couple of times a year, as I did when I was growing up, those extra calories won't affect your weight. If you eat at a restaurant two or more times a week, however, the extra calories will affect your weight unless you take some precautions. For John and me, Sunday afternoons were a favorite time to take the kids to a restaurant. Sometimes the many steps required to get the children fed and dressed in their Sunday clothes and looking fresh and neat for church left me exhausted. After all that effort, when John asked if I'd like to eat out after church, I always said yes.

In today's society, going out to eat is as normal as brushing your teeth. In fact, when we tell people that we rarely eat out now, they greet us with shocked glances and exclamations of, "You're kidding!" Most people I know eat out on a fairly consistent basis. Whereas thirty years ago, wives were often home and had time to prepare meals, today a majority of women work outside the home, so it is understandably difficult to prepare healthy meals every day. Not impossible, but difficult. Since Americans do eat out so frequently and aren't likely to change that habit, we need to fight the temptation to think of every restaurant meal as a treat and a time to overindulge.

Years ago, when I was a consultant for Pampered Chef, I began home sales parties by asking guests how they felt about cooking. I got a variety of responses, but one of the most memorable was this: "I hate cooking. The only time I ever cook is when I don't have enough money to go out to eat." The room erupted with laughter, but privately I agreed with the speaker. At the time, I didn't like to cook very much either, so anytime we had extra money, I'd willingly spend it on a restaurant meal. When I started losing weight, I did not stop eating out, but I did take the time to examine why I enjoyed eating out so often.

Your Turn

What is your favorite meal to eat out? Breakfast, lunch, dinner, or brunch?

_____

_____

Why that particular meal? _____

_____

_____

How often do you eat that meal out? _____

_____

When you eat at a restaurant you are familiar with, do you
usually know what you will have ahead of time?...................... Yes ❑ No ❑

On what do you base your selection? _____

_____

_____

How often do you frequent restaurants with buffets or drive-through windows? _____

_____

_____

Do you do a good job controlling your food intake while
dining at those types of restaurants?... Yes ❑ No ❑

Why or why not? _____

_____

_____

How many calories do you think are in your favorite restaurant meal?

_____

_____

List all the reasons you can think of for eating in restaurants: _____

_____

_____

Do you think it's possible to lose weight, maintain a healthy
weight, and still eat out frequently? .... Yes ❑ No ❑

Why or why not? _____

_____

_____

_____

How many times a week, including breakfast, lunch, and dinner, do you eat out? _____

_____

_____

What is your favorite restaurant? _____

_____

_____

How many times during an average week do you cook meals at home?

Breakfast: _____
Lunch: _____
Dinner: _____

Why? _____

_____

_____

_____

Restaurant Food Is Just Plain Food

Although many of us eat out a lot, we still think of it as a treat. Therefore, when we do go out, we tend to eat differently than we do at home. Do you find this to be true? How do you feel when you look at your favorite restaurant menu? Do you feel you are there for a treat or a special occasion and not solely to satisfy your body's natural desire and need for food?

Because we tend to treat each restaurant meal like a special occasion, we unintentionally give ourselves mental permission to gorge. That is how I operated all the years I was overweight. It didn't matter what restaurant we went to. I eagerly looked forward to sitting down and selecting my food. It was even more fun to go to a new restaurant. I could just feel the anticipation and excitement building as we walked to our seats. I just knew this was going to be great. Sometimes the food was great, and sometimes it wasn't, but I could always count on getting the entrée that promised the most food.

You read that right. I chose my entrée based on *quantity* rather than *quality*. If we had never been to the restaurant before, I'd look around as we were walking to our table, scanning the other diners' plates for potential choices. *Oh*, I'd think, *That man's plate looks very full.* Or, *Look at her with just a salad. Who is she kidding?* By the time we made it to the table, I had an idea what I'd like to order—whatever the big man over there had! When the server came to our table, one of the first questions I'd ask was what side dishes came with the entrées. I was especially happy if in addition to side dishes, the meal came with free bread, chips, or some other extra food.

After placing our order, John and I would settle in to enjoy the extra food that invariably arrived before the entrees. Bread for you? Yes. Would you like more chips? Yes. More bread? Yes. Would you like to pay ninety-nine cents extra for some cheese dip? Yes. Honestly, we ate enough before dinner that we should have just gotten up and gone home right then. Our calorie count for our dinner meal was already off the charts. Of course, we didn't leave but stayed to eat all of our dinner, plus more of the extra food. When our plates were empty, the obese person's favorite question came from the server's mouth, "Can I bring you some dessert?"

I would look at John, he'd look at me, and we'd say, "Well, maybe. What do you have?" Spilling forth from the server's mouth came an array of delectable dessert choices. The server would await our decision. John would say, "Well, we could share the cobbler." At the same time, I would say, "I'd rather have Death by Chocolate." We'd each order our own dessert and promptly eat the whole thing. Time after time, we visited restaurants, new and old, seeking culinary delights of the largest size. Fortunately for John, his weight has never been out of control and this bad habit didn't affect him the way it did me.

Buffet restaurants, with their unlimited entrées, breads, and desserts, were heaven to me. After filling my plate a couple times, I'd start to feel embarrassed about getting up for more food, so I'd send John to get me another muffin or several more cookies, and he would reluctantly oblige. Buffet restaurants are slippery slopes for overeaters. On a typical breakfast buffet, for instance, you find some healthy choices, such as fresh fruit, cereal, or scrambled eggs, but you also find gigantic muffins, greasy sausages and bacon, biscuits laden with fat, French toast, and fried hash browns. When you look at this list, you might say to yourself, "Well, I'll just choose the more healthy foods." But if you are like most people, you'll probably make some good choices and lots of bad choices.

Is it difficult to eat the proper portions of healthy food when faced with so many choices? *Difficult* doesn't even begin to describe it. After I started changing my eating habits, I ordered meals off the menu. I found it interesting that servers tried to discourage me from doing so, saying, "Oh, you don't want two pancakes and an order of fruit. You can just get that on the buffet." The servers were right, but that wasn't what I wanted to do. I wanted to be in control of my portion sizes and to not have the potential for unlimited food choices. I discovered that one plate of food is enough for anyone. No one needs unlimited food for breakfast, lunch, or dinner. But many people have conditioned themselves to eat beyond the point of fullness.

Your Turn

Do you ever overeat at a restaurant? .... Yes ❑ No ❑

Do you typically eat more at a restaurant than you would
at home? .... Yes ❑ No ❑

Why or why not? _____

_____

_____

_____

What role does money play in the amount of food you eat at a restaurant?

_____

_____

Cheap Food

Buffets are hard on the waistline, but other types of restaurants are just as dangerous. All-you-can-eat specials are a dime a dozen, and like the popular sandwich commercial used to say, "Fat is cheap." Restaurants advertise their various ninety-nine-cent menus relentlessly. What do they feature on those menus? Fried hamburgers, French-fried potatoes, fried onion rings, sugar-filled drinks, fat-laden pork biscuits, and high-calorie milkshakes. To be fair, some restaurants do offer a small salad or fruit cup as part of the ninety-nine-cent menu, but when I was overweight, given the choice between a juicy, filling hamburger or some iceberg lettuce with a mealy tomato, I'd choose the hamburger every time.

What do restaurants have to gain by offering such inexpensive items, especially considering the rising cost of goods and services? A loyal following. They want us to visit their establishments and keep coming back, and they willingly take a loss on certain items to ensure we comply. Most restaurants don't care about our weight or our health. They want our business. Keep that in mind when you see inexpensive food advertised on television. Catchy slogans, colorful billboards, revolving signs, and cheap food are all marketing gimmicks, and they usually involve unhealthy food choices.

My weight in college was normal, although it did creep up a bit over the four years once I started shunning the college cafeteria in favor of the fast-food havens near campus. When John and I married, we both enjoyed fast food and ate it many times a week. These journeys into the fast-food world were rarely, if ever, planned, and neither of us gave any serious thought to the healthiness or calorie content of the foods we chose. As poor newlyweds, we saw fast food as an inexpensive option for dining out. Both of us could eat for $6 and still have money left for ice cream at Dairy Queen!

The perceived value of fast food is high. The food is delivered fast, it is readily available, it's consistent (a Big Mac at the McDonald's across town will taste the same as a Big Mac in your neighborhood), and it's cheap. You can even "value size" or "supersize" the meal for just a few pennies more.

I loved ordering a double cheeseburger value meal, supersized of course. I used to justify supersizing by reminding myself that I wanted a large drink, and the easiest way to get the large drink was to have the large fries too. Fast-food restaurants became my secret food oases, places I could go to satisfy my emotional and physical cravings for high-fat food on a budget.

I found myself pulling into the drive-through when I was bored, stressed, or upset—and then lying to John about what I had done. Occasionally, after I made a covert run through a drive-through, I picked up John or the kids from an event. Having already thrown away the offending bags, I would happily pull up to get them. John would get in the car and say, "It smells like hamburgers in here." I would look blankly at that man, as if to say, "I don't have the faintest idea what you are talking about!" Even the older children could tell if I'd had something tasty in the car. They would say, "Did you save us any fries, Mommy?" Again, I'd just shake my head in a way that would let them know they were mistaken. I still feel bad about lying to my family.

The instant comfort of high-fat, cheap food, combined with twenty-four-hour-a-day availability, makes fast food hard to resist. I fell prey to the lure of those restaurants, and if the astronomical success of restaurant chains is any indication, I wasn't alone.

Your Turn

Do you ever impulsively stop at a certain fast-food
restaurant? .... Yes ❑ No ❑

Why that particular restaurant? _____
_____
_____

Under what circumstances? _____
_____
_____

What do you typically order? _____
_____
_____

Have you ever been dishonest about food you purchased
at a fast-food restaurant? .... Yes ❑ No ❑

What were the circumstances? _____
_____
_____

Can you commit to not lying about what you eat.................. Yes ❑ No ❑

Sit-Down Restaurants

I'd like to share a story about a restaurant I loved to visit when I was a big girl. We were living in Florida. The "free" food at this restaurant was a bucketful of peanuts, and patrons could discard empty shells on the floor. The restaurant was perfect for our family. It was loud, it was already dirty, and the kids' meals were popular with my children.

I share this story to illustrate how out of control my eating habits were and how with some hard work and diligence they changed. On this particular evening, we had the two girls with us, and the server asked if we would like a table or a booth. A booth, we both replied. As we followed her around to our appointed booth, I was mentally measuring the space between the booth and the table to make sure I would fit. I was pretty sure I would. I hopped up on the step and tried to squeeze myself into the booth. I didn't quite fit, but that didn't stop me. I just squeezed a little harder. As the booth creaked slightly, I popped in—never to get out until dinner was over. I was so squished that I could hardly breathe. It felt like my entire upper body was resting on the tabletop. Quite embarrassing, but the polite waitress didn't say a word and just asked what drinks she could bring. "Diet Coke for me," I said.

During the meal, I ate at least half a bucket of peanuts, which was probably enough calories for the day right there, and that was even before the main meal arrived. Bless that server's heart, because she also brought us the restaurant's famous yeast rolls. I ate three or four yeast rolls smothered in butter, finished off my huge chicken sandwich and my baked potato with butter and sour cream, and then proceeded to eat left-over food from the girls' plates. I remember sitting at that booth feeling unbelievably full and disgusted with myself for eating so much food. But I wasn't done yet. I popped myself out of the booth, waddled out of the restaurant, and helped John load the girls into the car. We then looked at each other and said, "You want dessert?" We drove right across the street to the ice cream shop and ordered large cones—one dipped in chocolate for me and one dipped in butterscotch for John. By rights, I should have been sick after all that, but I had trained my body to eat large amounts of food, and although I was uncomfortable, I wasn't ill.

Now perhaps you haven't been that gluttonous. Perhaps you have. Estimates show that when eating out, people tend to consume an average of 300 more calories per meal than normal.

Your Turn

What restaurant foods do you eat in excess? _____

_____

_____

Why do these foods tempt you? _____

_____

_____

We Have a Choice

We can bash restaurants all we want, but they aren't to blame. They are just offering a service, and we as consumers have a choice to take advantage of that service or not. However, the food selections at most restaurants aren't generally conducive to healthy eating making it difficult to make healthy choices. It often requires advanced planning and willingness to set yourself apart from other diners at your table.

You may be wondering whether we stopped going out to eat once I began to change my eating habits. When I began following my plan, I realized right away that I needed to do the things I loved, and that included going out to eat. Just because I changed my eating habits, I didn't stop doing things I enjoyed. It wasn't practical for me to say, "I'm on a diet. I can't go out to eat."

Since I've been teaching the Fit to the Finish class, I've known several people who stopped going out to eat because they felt they couldn't control their portion sizes at restaurants. One friend, who was following another diet plan, chose not to go out to eat until she reached her desired weight-loss goal of 20 pounds. Once she finally achieved her goal, she began going out to eat again, but because she hadn't changed her lifestyle and attitude toward food, she gained back all the weight she had lost, plus a little more, within three months.

Like me, you can continue to eat out and still lose weight, and when you achieve your weight-loss goal, you can still eat out and maintain your healthy weight. It's much easier to eat out on a weight-loss plan now than it was years ago. When I was losing weight, restaurants that offered low-fat, low-calorie entrées were few and far between. Now it's the rare restaurant that doesn't offer at least a few "light fare" choices.

Each meal you eat on the Fit to the Finish plan can take you one step closer to achieving your weight-loss goal. Every snack, every breakfast, and, yes, every meal eaten away from home gives you the same opportunity. When you are dining out, it's vital to make the most healthful selection you can.

Your Turn

When looking at a restaurant menu, do you notice whether it lists low-fat entrees? .... Yes ❑ No ❑

Why or why not? _____

_____

_____

If they are listed, do you select one? .... Yes ❑ No ❑

Why or why not? _____

_____

_____

Study the Menu

When I was heavy, I liked my meals big and abundant. When I started losing weight, I realized that restaurant meals were bigger and more abundant than even I, a 300-pound woman, needed. Restaurant portions have gotten so out of sync with anything that even resembles a healthy meal that it's almost laughable. Restaurant portion sizes began increasing in the 1970s and ballooned out of control in the 1980s and 1990s. Once we as consumers became accustomed to large portions, there was no going back. So if larger portions are here to stay, what can you do?

It's not impossible to lose weight and go out to eat frequently, but it does require preplanning and a commitment to going against the tide.

There is no reason not to choose the lower-fat, lower-calorie entrées at restaurants whether you are dieting or not. Some menus have little "healthy" symbols by meals that are low in fat and calories. Other menus have "Healthy Choices" or "Lite Fare" sections. In many cases, vegetarian and vegan entrées are by default healthy. A vegetarian entrée uses no meat but may include cheese or eggs. A vegan entrée uses no animal products at all, including butter, cheese, milk, or eggs. Plant-based entrees are generally lower in saturated fats and have fewer calories. Select a meal with the least amount of fat and salt possible and then eat only what you know to be a proper portion. Ask to substitute certain components. If the entrée includes fries, ask the server if you can have steamed vegetables, a baked potato, or side salad instead of the fries. Although the ingredient list will likely not be available for many restaurant meals, learn to identify healthy and unhealthy items on restaurant menus. Avoid entrées or side dishes that are fried, have fatty cuts of beef, or have large amounts of cheese or sauce.

Play Twenty Questions with the Server

What do you do if the restaurant you're at doesn't cater to your dietary needs? It takes a little planning, and often a little nerve, but restaurants will work with you concerning the preparation of your food.

I'm not a very assertive person by nature, so this approach took some practice for me. It was especially difficult when I first started following my plan, because I often wondered what the server was thinking. Here's the scenario: An obese woman walks into a restaurant with her husband. They request to be seated at a table rather than a booth because the woman is worried she may not fit into a booth. Upon being asked what she would like to eat, the fat woman proceeds to question the server about the preparation of the food. Are those vegetables sautéed in oil? Is the pasta cooked with oil in the water? Is the chicken coated with butter before it's grilled? Is the bun large or small?

I often wondered what the server thought of me right then. How odd it must have been to wait on a woman who was obviously not in shape but was meticulous about how her food was prepared. I never had a server who wasn't gracious and accommodating. Every single waitperson was willing to help me figure out what a good choice would be. And these days, with the number of people suffering from food allergies and sensitivities, servers are accustomed to patrons inquiring about specific ingredients and preparation.

Because I learned to be assertive, I made good choices and lost weight in the process. I enjoy meals out with my family, knowing I am not over-eating, and I love leaving the restaurant without feeling guilty.

Premeal Food: Just Say No

Another aspect of restaurant eating, particularly in sit-down restaurants, is premeal food—the bread, chips and salsa, peanuts, or other foods meant to keep you from getting overly hungry and irritable before your server delivers your meal. When it comes to premeal food, I have some words for you: "No thank-you." That's it. You don't need to think about it. You just need to refuse it. All premeal food does is fill you up with calories you should be eating at your actual meal.

The first time I looked a server straight in the eye and said "No thank-you" to premeal food, John looked at me as if I had lost my mind. What was I thinking?

I told John, "I'm so sorry, but I just can't have those yeast rolls sitting on the table winking at me." He was a little disappointed, but because he wanted me to be successful, he suffered alongside me.

The premeal food situation can be a bit difficult if you are dining with someone other than family members or close friends. Work associates or casual acquaintances may take offense at your decision to refuse premeal food for the entire table. In those situations, put a piece of gum in your mouth and chew away. This will keep your mouth occupied with something other than food until your meal comes along.

Occasionally, someone at the table would ask why I wasn't having any chips. I'd just say, "I don't care for any right now." That was the end of the discussion. No awkward moments; no weird feelings. I realized that any perceived awkwardness was in my head and that my dinner companions didn't care whether I was eating chips. After all, the less I ate, the more they could have.

Order First

The server comes to the table, looks around, and asks, "Are you ready to order?" In my fat days, I always wanted to order last, so if someone chose something that looked better than what I had initially selected, I could change my mind at the very last minute. Let me give you a tip: be assertive. You've already made your decision, so go ahead and order first.

By ordering first, you take the pressure off yourself to be swayed by what others are having. Even if the server doesn't look directly at you when he or she asks for your table's order, just pipe up and say, "I'm ready." And then stick with your plan. In the past, if I realized that my friend was going to have the big platter of fried chicken wings, I felt that gave me permission to order the big platter too. After all, if she was going to eat like a pig, I could too.

The concept works both ways. Once I started losing weight and ordering healthier foods, my friends would say, "Oh, you're going to be good? Well, maybe I should have the salad too." They sometimes looked disappointed, because they felt compelled to make a healthy choice as well. Fat loves company—but so do healthy choices. So order first!

Portion Your Own Food

Starting now, when you go out to eat, make the healthiest choice you can by ordering a low-fat entrée and sides, by asking that your food be baked or grilled instead of fried, or by requesting that no butter be added to the meal. These simple choices will help you stay on track for your eating plan that day. Now that you've avoided the premeal food and ordered wisely, you can enjoy your meal guilt-free—almost. There's one more thing: You still need to watch portion sizes. Portion sizes for low-fat entrées at restaurants are generally appropriate. But if your meal arrives and you can see that the portion is too large, you need to move the offending amount either to the side of your plate or into a takeout box. You can still unintentionally consume too many calories by eating too much of a good thing.

If you have ordered a standard entrée, you will definitely need to adjust your portion size. A good rule of thumb is to eat half or less of the portion the restaurant serves you. Another strategy is to split a meal with a dining buddy. Most restaurants accommodate this request, although some charge a small fee for doing so.

Why do most of us feel the need to eat our entire entrée at a restaurant when we don't feel the same compulsion at home? My theory is that at home, you aren't thinking about the money it cost you to make the meal. You are focusing on your dining companions and keeping the children happy, and when you are full, you stop. At a restaurant, we want to get the best value for our money, and many people think the only way to achieve that is to eat the whole thing.

In truth, the meal is only as valuable as it is good for you. It's not a good value if you eat the whole plate and blow your calorie allotment for the day. Portion control isn't always easy, but it is always worth the good feeling you'll have when you leave the restaurant.

I now look at restaurant meals differently. I no longer think of a dining experience as a reward for a long day at work or as a treat (unless it's my anniversary or Valentine's Day). I look at an everyday restaurant meal as just that—a meal, plain and simple. The next time you go out to eat, view your meal with this new philosophy. It will give you permission not to clear your plate.

Your Turn

Do you typically eat all of your entrée when dining out?......... Yes ❏ No ❏

At home, do you always clean your plate? .... Yes ❏ No ❏

If your answers are different, explain the difference:

_____

_____

_____

15

Pregnancy Quadrupled

I never had a 75-pound baby, but I did have a 75-pound pregnancy. The normal recommended weight gain for pregnant women is between 25 and 35 pounds. Even if I had been carrying triplets, 75 pounds would have been too much (the average weight gain for triplets is about 60 pounds). I wasn't carrying multiple babies, just one little 8-pound baby girl. And after her birth, I was one really large, squishy, exhausted mom.

After Rachel was born, I lost a miniscule amount of weight and never lost any more pregnancy fat. Three years later, when I got pregnant for the second time, my beginning weight was 255 pounds. I experienced the shame and humiliation of having the doctor see my floppy belly, felt exhausted from day 1 of the pregnancy to day 270, and was embarrassed every time I stood on the scale. The entire trip to the doctor's office was spent with me internally coaching myself on the necessity of being weighed, while at the same time reminding myself that the doctor had seen lots of fat pregnant people in his long career.

With my second and third pregnancies, I was so fat that I looked pregnant before I got pregnant. Friends and acquaintances who didn't know I was expecting couldn't tell by just looking at me. It wasn't until I was about six months pregnant that people finally started noticing something different about my appearance. Believe me, I wasn't about to wear a T-shirt with an arrow pointing to my stomach with the message "Baby Aboard." In fact, I hardly needed to buy maternity clothes because my jumpers were made for large abdomens. I had purposefully made them with some built-in growing room, just in case I gained weight. And gain weight I did.

The Risks of Obesity in Pregnancy

I was fortunate that I went through three pregnancies at an obese weight without any complications. However, obesity in pregnancy carries many real risks.

Obese mothers have a higher likelihood of requiring a cesarean section. Although cesarean deliveries are routinely performed, the surgery still has risks, especially for an obese mother. She might develop blood clots or suffer severe blood loss. The incision might not heal properly. She might be left with scars that remain painful long after they have healed.

A pregnant woman whose weight places her in the obese range is also at a higher risk for developing gestational diabetes, according to the Centers for Disease Control and Prevention. Additionally, if you are obese, your child is two times more likely to develop type 2 diabetes. Uncontrolled gestational diabetes increases the risk of your baby getting too large, which can lead to shoulder dystocia, a situation in which the baby's shoulders get stuck in your birth canal during delivery. This emergency can cause brain damage or death to the baby from a lack of oxygen, result in long-term arm and shoulder problems, or result in a broken collarbone during delivery. If you are diabetic and your blood sugar levels are not properly controlled through diet and/or medications, your baby could also develop low blood sugar shortly after birth. Every time I took a diabetes test during pregnancy, I was very worried. My midwife was surprised I never developed it.

Blood pressure problems are also more common in pregnant obese women, perhaps because being obese naturally increases your risk of high blood pressure. Fetal death is also a risk for obese pregnant women, as reported in a 2011 study in the journal *Human Reproduction*. According to the study, beginning a pregnancy at an obese weight almost doubles the risk of the baby dying either during the pregnancy or up to twelve months later. Preeclampsia, which is the development of high blood pressure and the presence of protein in a pregnant woman's urine, is likely responsible for a portion of the increased risk of fetal death in obese women.

If you do begin a pregnancy while you are overweight, talk to your doctor about an appropriate weight gain for your situation. Your doctor may request that you consult with a nutritionist to help with calorie intake and food choices.

One evening at church, an acquaintance asked me, "Diane, someone said you are pregnant. Is that true?" I nodded and told her that I was in fact thirty-two weeks along. That's right. I was so fat that my friend, a mom of five herself, couldn't tell I was pregnant at thirty-two weeks. She was embarrassed, I was embarrassed, and we both stood there and looked awkwardly at each other. I finally made a joke of it. I rubbed my stomach and said, "I guess I'm just carrying the baby really low." We laughed together, but inside I felt like crying.

After my second daughter was born, I lost some weight and got down to a four-year low of 224 pounds. I had worked hard at making better food choices and was proud of myself for being closer to 200 pounds than to 250. But I got complacent, life got complicated, and I got fat again. I was once again eating M&M's like they were the last food on earth, consuming entire family-size bags of chips, and sitting on the couch all day long like a big lump. I sank into depression over the sad state of my life and ate in a fruitless attempt to make myself feel better.

Day after day, I'd promise myself not to overeat. I had been 224 pounds for one day; I could be 224 pounds again. But instead, the scale showed a steady increase. I know at my highest I weighed at least 305 pounds. It could have been more though. My bathroom scale had a capacity of 300 pounds, and that scale maxed out on me. Therefore, the only way I saw 305 pounds on a scale, other than at the doctor's office, was when I jumped on a gigantic scale in the grocery story lobby late one night. The long dial swung around to 305 and I jumped off, looking around to make sure no one had seen the number.

After that jump on the scale, I panicked and actually lost a few pounds. And you know what happened next? I got pregnant for the third time. My starting weight was 279. I was mortified at my first visit to the doctor and braced myself for the usual, "You really should watch your weight during this pregnancy, Diane." My doctor was very nice and never made me feel bad about myself. My thoughts did that without him saying a word.

I dreaded my monthly appointments, not only because of the required weigh-ins but also because I had to expose my belly to the doctor and nurse. I'd lie back on the table and keep my shirt down until the last possible second. Then the doctor would say, "Let's listen to the baby's heartbeat." He'd look at me expectantly, and I'd lift up my shirt so he could find the heartbeat. It was thrilling to hear the baby, but overshadowing the excitement of a new life inside me was my mortification that my belly, thighs, and shoulders extended over the sides of the exam table. I still remember my doctor being unable to stand normally to place the fetal Doppler on my belly. Instead, he took a small step away from the table, bent forward a bit, and reached his arm over me to listen to the heartbeat.

Although I liked to hear the baby's heartbeat, I was anxious to cover up my pregnant belly when he was done. He'd wipe the gel off and I'd pull down my shirt, relieved everything was okay with the baby and glad I didn't have to show my belly for another few weeks.

Every appointment brought unnecessary weight gain. Mid-pregnancy arrived, and I scheduled an appointment to have the standard twenty-week ultrasound. I was excited to see the baby on the ultrasound monitor but even more excited to find out whether I was carrying a boy. We had two daughters and longed for a son. This pregnancy felt different from my first two. I just had a feeling the baby was a boy.

The morning of the scheduled appointment finally arrived. John and I left the girls with a friend and drove to the doctor's office. Although I was eagerly anticipating the ultrasound, I wasn't very excited about having to show my oversized pregnant belly to anyone, especially when I saw the fit young technician who called us back.

I waddled down the hallway and all of a sudden started experiencing a lot of apprehension. What would the technician think of my gigantic belly when I lay on the table? She had to touch it. John would see it. I kept waddling, trying to focus on seeing the baby and not seeing my belly.

I lay on the exam table and pulled up my shirt. There it was in all its white, stretch-marked glory: a twenty-week pregnant belly on an almost-300-pound beached whale. I was glad the lights were dim, but that didn't dim my embarrassment. The tech squirted half a bottle of gel on my belly and began the ultrasound. I was extremely self-conscious when she asked me to pull on the top of my abdomen so she could get a better picture, but I obliged her request. My arms got tired holding up the weight of my stomach, but it was worth the discomfort to have a clearer picture of the baby.

It was fun to see all the baby parts, and I couldn't wait to hear her say, "It's a . . ." She pointed out the head, the heart, the stomach, and the legs, but she didn't say the gender. Finally, I asked her, "Can you tell what the baby is?" She pressed the transducer more firmly over my belly and looked hard at the monitor. She shook her head.

"I'm just not sure," she said. She looked again, this time moving the transducer to a different angle. It felt like she was pushing that thing all the way to my backbone. She shook her head again. "I'm sorry. I don't want to say unless I'm 100 percent certain, and I just can't get a clear picture."

"Oh," I said. "Is the baby in a bad position?"

She hesitated but finally explained. "It's not the baby's position but rather the amount of abdominal fat you have." I could tell she didn't want to say those words, but I had asked. I looked at her, not knowing what to say. So I let her words lie there alone. Even though I didn't say anything, I felt shattered. I struggled to continue listening to her soothing words.

She hastened to explain that if we came back in six weeks, the baby would be bigger, and it would be easier to tell the gender in spite of the abdominal fat. I nodded solemnly. After she wiped all the gel off my squishy belly, I worked my way off the table. John and I walked silently back to the appointment desk, where we made another appointment six weeks in the future.

The car ride back to John's office was a little bit subdued. I had been so excited about the ultrasound, and although I was thrilled that the tech didn't see any problems with the baby, I was less than thrilled about the abdominal fat comment. John wisely didn't say anything about her comment but rather tried to cheer me up by talking about how cute the baby had been on the monitor and how much fun it would be to have another ultrasound in six weeks. I grunted at him and tried to be a little cheery. I failed.

After I dropped him off at work, but before I went and picked up the girls, I went to the drive-through at Chick-fil-A and bought a large combo meal and a dessert. I ate all that food as fast as I could, trying in vain to stuff the bad emotions down with bad-for-me food.

Six weeks passed, and the next ultrasound appointment was short and uneventful. I still experienced the humiliation of having to expose my belly to the world, but I was rewarded by finding out that the baby was definitely a boy. I was over the moon.

The rest of the pregnancy passed slowly. I thoroughly enjoyed preparing the nursery and buying tiny blue clothes. It was fun to imagine that our baby would soon be wearing the impossibly tiny sleepers and onesies. But as fun as the baby prep was, being pregnant at almost 300 pounds was absolutely exhausting. It was all I could do to get through my day. I took frequent naps, sat on the couch as much as possible, and avoided any kind of physical activity. I couldn't wait for Mark to be born.

Finally, on our tenth wedding anniversary, Mark arrived. Baby weighed 8 pounds 13 ounces, and Mom was way above 300 pounds. He was precious, and I was so relieved that he was healthy in spite of my obesity. I once again experienced the shame of being an obese hospital patient and couldn't wait to go home with my new baby. In spite of my discomfort, I understood how blessed I was that my weight hadn't affected him in a negative way.

I loved having another baby but felt the weight of my obesity more than ever. Even after recovering from the birth, I had no energy, wasn't losing weight, and felt horrible about myself.

At a routine doctor's visit some months after Mark's birth, I had the "aha moment" that began my last weight-loss journey. In the fourteen months following that appointment, I lost 150 pounds and regained my life. I conquered fear, conquered horrible eating habits, and enjoyed a level of fitness I had never known.

Then it happened. I got pregnant again. And I miscarried. I got pregnant again. And I miscarried again. I remember asking my doctor if the weight loss had anything to do with two miscarriages in a row. He reassured

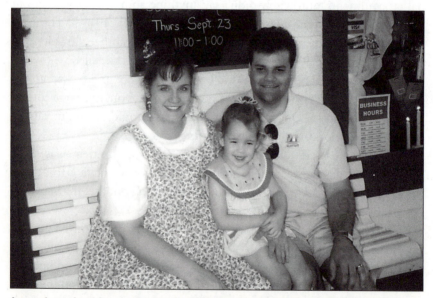

I was hot, tired, and extremely irritable at this point in my pregnancy. Seeing how awful I looked in this picture made me want to throw the camera in the trash.

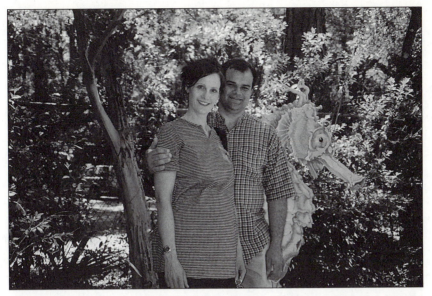

Even I was surprised when I saw this picture of John and myself. I had a hard time believing I could be pregnant without looking like a beached whale.

me that if anything, pregnancies would be easier and less prone to complications at a healthier weight. I remember saying to him, "I'd rather be fat and have those babies I lost than be thin and continually miscarry." Saddened beyond words after the miscarriages, John and I talked at length about whether to try again. We prayed about it and felt there was still another baby for us. So, with some trepidation, we got pregnant again.

This time the pregnancy looked healthy from the beginning. The fear of miscarriage subsided as the weeks went by, but the fear of extraordinary weight gain began to enter my mind. My fears were unfounded. During my fourth full-term pregnancy, I gained only 29 pounds.

Compare the picture of me at eight months pregnant with my second baby (page 190) to the picture of me (*above*) at seven months pregnant with my fourth child and note the incredible difference in my appearance.

But the differences went far beyond my appearance. Yes, for the first time I gained an appropriate amount of weight in a pregnancy, but I also experienced some psychological differences that I attribute to being pregnant at a healthier weight.

Changes in Attitude

During my first three pregnancies, I used my condition as an excuse to eat anything I wanted, anytime I wanted, in any quantity I wanted. I ate enough fruits, vegetables, and proteins for four people, rather than just for me and a tiny, growing baby. I ate not only three large meals each day but also all the snacks, sweets, and ice cream I wanted.

I went into the fourth pregnancy with a completely different attitude toward food. My doctor told me that gaining between 25 and 35 pounds would be appropriate, and I agreed with him. So I stopped using pregnancy as an excuse to pull my chair up to the feed bucket and eat for nine solid months. Instead, I planned my meals carefully and paid attention to quantity as well as quality.

Like many women, I suffered from all-day sickness during the first trimester. With my first three pregnancies, I had grazed on whatever sounded good in a vain attempt to keep the nausea at bay. It didn't work. Instead of the nausea going away, I only made it worse with my food choices. Sure, tomato and mayonnaise sandwiches sounded good initially, but after I was done eating that, I'd wish I hadn't even begun. And then, because I felt worse than before, I'd try some chips and dip. All day long, I'd jump from one food to another, using my nausea as an excuse.

The fourth pregnancy was no different than the first three with regard to my level of nausea. If anything, it was a little worse. I had learned my lesson about extreme weight gain but needed some new strategies to help with the nausea. I knew that junk food didn't make me feel better, so I drank slightly flavored water, ate a few crackers before I got out of bed, kept healthy fruits and veggies in the refrigerator, sucked on hard candy, drank peppermint tea, and prayed for relief.

Did any of these strategies get rid of the nausea? No. But neither did eating huge quantities of food all day long. I still gained a few pounds during the first trimester, but that was normal and healthy. And when the nausea finally passed, I wasn't already up 20 pounds as I had been in previous pregnancies. What a blessing!

During the last six months of the pregnancy, I ate like a normal pregnant woman, adding in the 300 extra calories per day recommended for pregnancy. One of the many things I had learned during my weight-loss journey was that calories add up quickly. Three hundred calories was about the equivalent of two slices of bread, a thin spreading of peanut butter, and an apple. *That's it.*

Honestly, it took some adjustments to be satisfied with eating like a healthy pregnant person rather than an obese pregnant person. It was still tempting to use my pregnancy as an excuse for "free eating." But instead of free eating, I enjoyed eating in freedom. I was free to eat those foods that were good for both the baby and me. I made sure to eat the right amounts and not overindulge day after day. And it worked.

I felt one hundred times better during my fourth pregnancy than I had during the first three pregnancies. I had more energy, I slept better, and I looked better. And as an added bonus, even labor was easier. I was induced with the fourth pregnancy and within four hours was holding my sweet baby Noah. I still remember one of the nurses walking in after I had just given birth and saying, "Look at you, skinny." Of course, I wasn't skinny, but neither was I the 260-pound obese whale I had been before.

My recovery was a piece of cake compared to the other pregnancies. I fit into my bigger jeans within two weeks.

Within six to eight weeks, I had lost all my pregnancy weight and could fit into most of my regular clothes. And I didn't diet during those six weeks. Rather, I ate appropriately, all the while mindful of the fact that I was nursing. Although each person is different, my doctor recommended that I eat at least 2,000 calories while I was nursing, which would allow me to lose weight and still properly nourish the baby.

That fourth pregnancy was an eye-opening experience for me. The difference between an obese pregnancy and an average-weight pregnancy is astounding. It was almost as if I had lived two separate lives—before obesity and after. But within the joy and ease of that pregnancy, I felt some pangs of sadness for how I had treated my body before I lost all my weight. I had to work through some of those regretful feelings while moving forward to enjoy my second son.

I began exercising after my six-week checkup by simply walking. I listened to my body's cues and moved slowly at first. As I felt stronger and more energetic, I strove to once again go faster and farther. There were days when John had to leave for work earlier than I could exercise, so when those days came around, I took all four children walking with me. I'd put the two little boys in the stroller. The girls, then ages ten and seven, would ride their bikes 3.5 miles. We all enjoyed the trips, especially the girls. Sometimes when they woke up and found I had already exercised, they were disappointed, so I'd take them out later in the day.

Subsequent Pregnancies

I wish I could say that pregnancies five, six, and seven were as picture perfect as number four, but I can't. I did gain more weight than I should have with those last three pregnancies. I could list every excuse I gave myself for gaining 40 pounds or more, but I won't. Instead, I'll tell you that I had back problems that limited my movement, was sick long beyond the first trimester, and was fearful of miscarriage. So I sat more than I normally did and ate more too.

I didn't eat bad foods, but I ate more healthy foods than I needed to. My doctors were never concerned with my weight gain. Despite the weight gain and other issues, my last three pregnancies were still far easier than my first three obese pregnancies.

After each birth, I continued following my Fit to the Finish weight-loss plan. I ate small portions of healthy food to control my calorie intake and drop the pregnancy pounds. I watched the percentage of fats in foods and exercised when I received my doctor's okay. I would be lying if I said I wasn't frustrated with myself after each of those pregnancies, when I had to lose some weight all over again. But I knew I could get back down to a size 6. Why was I so confident? Because I had already lost 150 pounds once before, and I had a plan that worked. I knew I could count on success if I followed everything in the Fit to the Finish plan.

I always took my time losing weight after the babies were born. I was a nursing mother, which meant I needed to eat more calories to make certain the baby received enough nutrients. I didn't cut back my calories to an extreme level; nor did I exercise myself into oblivion. With each of the last three pregnancies, it took between four and six months to get back down to my healthy weight. I focused on the baby and my family while still being mindful of my weight and health.

My doctors, who were aware of my history, were pleased with me at my six-week checkups and just encouraged me to eat good foods and exercise. When I saw them again for my annual exam, I was back down to my ideal weight. It was a good feeling to go into the doctor's office, stand on the scale, and not feel like running away. I didn't like standing on the scale, but it didn't frighten me and make me want to eat ice cream either.

Body after Pregnancy

Very few women can have a few babies and look exactly like they did pre-pregnancy. I couldn't. Perhaps if I had never been obese or had one child instead of seven, I could have. But that wasn't my situation.

After the first three obese pregnancies, I didn't even try to get in shape because I hadn't been in shape in the first place. Instead of working to improve my appearance and figure, I just kept eating and thus made everything worse. I drooped in places that shouldn't droop. I bulged in places where no bulges should be, and I had a huge shelf hanging off my backside. What's a shelf?

Please allow me to explain. One day after I had lost 150 pounds, John and I were looking at some pictures. In those pictures I weighed close to 300 pounds and didn't look so good. I was pointing out various things, such as the tightness of my sleeves and the unstylish clothing, when he said, "And there's the shelf." I looked at him and said, "The what?"

He blushed and said, "Never mind." I insisted, and he reluctantly explained that when I was overweight, right below my waist was a body part he thought of as a shelf. It protruded out from the roundness of the rest of my body and sat there like a ledge. When I walked, it moved around as if independent from the rest of me. I instantly knew what he was talking about, as I had noticed the extra movement around my middle, but to realize that he had a name for it was astonishing. I wasn't sure if I should laugh or cry.

He told me that after every pregnancy, the shelf got a little bigger and more pronounced. Just to be clear, John was never critical of my weight and was always supportive and loving. I don't think he meant any harm. His casual phrase just slipped out without any malice. In some ways it was funny, and it some ways it was sad. But it certainly was honest.

And he was right. After each of the pregnancies, the shelf got a little larger—along with the rest of me. I made no attempt to exercise because I believed I would be too tired given all my other mom responsibilities. So I let the shelf get bigger and the rest of me get flabbier.

After the extreme weight loss and the fourth pregnancy, the last thing I wanted was to be flabby. So in addition to walking, running, and biking, I added in some strength training. I worked with light weights in my bedroom several times a week. Everything firmed up as much as it could, and I was satisfied with my appearance. I repeated this routine after each pregnancy because there was one thing I knew for sure: I did not want to see the shelf reappear.

The shelf made it almost impossible to fit into restaurant booths. The shelf made my shirts ride up no matter how many times I pulled them down. The shelf was heavy to haul around. Having been on both sides of the weight issue, I'd rather be living on the fit side than the fat side.

Pregnancy doesn't have to be the death knell for your efforts to get and stay healthy. You can gain the appropriate amount of weight and then lose it again. And if you have a pregnancy where your weight gain is less than stellar, as I did, it's okay. You can just follow my healthy eating plan and lose weight at a steady, healthy pace.

Some women have told me that they would like to have another child but are so afraid of the pregnancy weight gain that they'd rather adopt. If you feel that way, I encourage you to remember my story. I had four healthy-weight pregnancies and lost weight after all of them. You can too.

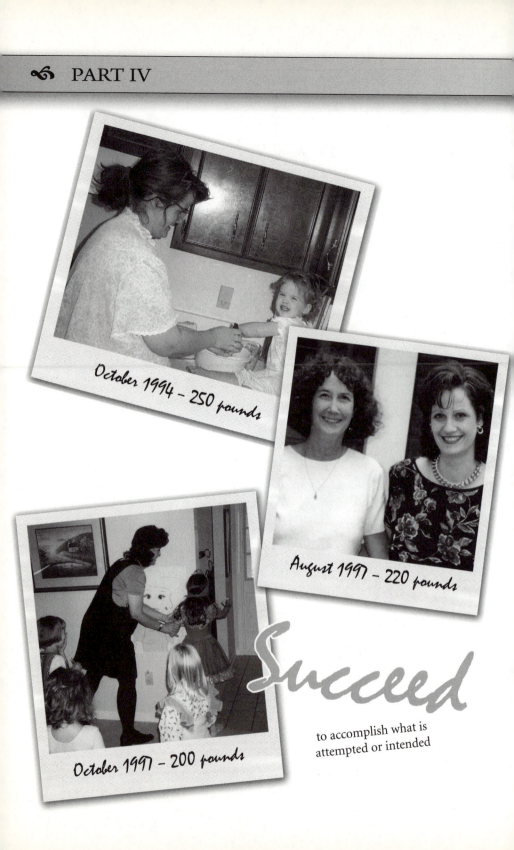

PART IV

October 1994 – 250 pounds

August 1997 – 220 pounds

October 1997 – 200 pounds

Succeed

to accomplish what is
attempted or intended

Beyond Weight Loss

N ow that you have completed the first three portions of the book, you may be wondering what comes next. The answer depends on how close you are to your weight-loss goal. If you are at your goal weight, you are ready to begin working on lifelong maintenance. If you still have pounds to lose, you are still ready to prepare for what lies beyond weight loss.

The maintenance portion of your journey is what you have worked so hard to achieve. As you read through the next two chapters, keep in mind that the techniques I share with you can be used for years to come. You may want to reread the chapters after you reach your goal weight to refresh your memory on how to handle this very exciting time of your life.

16

Planning for Success

Isn't it wonderful to begin shaping your weight-loss journey using the tools provided in this book? Can you imagine how amazing you will feel as you live the rest of your life fit and healthy? Picture participating in everything you desire and not letting your weight affect your choices in any way. That rosy scenario can occur only with your continued hard work and dedication to looking ahead with a firm plan.

As we continue our experience together, I would be remiss if I didn't dedicate a chapter to planning—not only meal planning but also planning for various holidays and special events. Let's talk about how to plan the meals that you and your family eat. Let's make a plan that you can live with for the rest of your life—one that is flexible enough to allow for life's inevitable changes and rigid enough to give you long-term success.

A Basic Principle

Planning seems like a basic principle, doesn't it? After all, we start planning our lives from the time we are small children. When I was five, I planned to be a ballerina. When I was ten, I thought I'd be a gymnast. When I was twelve, being a veterinarian held great appeal. As a teenager, I thought I would be a great clarinetist. As a student in college, Wall Street was my goal. As I have gotten older, I've realized that plans don't always pan out. I never dreamed, as a newly married young woman, that I'd have seven children and live in a small town. I also never planned or expected to be obese for ten years of my married life.

Your Turn

What were your early plans for yourself? _____
_____
_____

How did they change over the years? _____
_____
_____

Planning Is Part of Life

Planning is a natural and normal part of everyday life. Even mundane tasks require planning. Let's take something as seemingly easy as attending a concert. We'll assume that you are married and have two children in elementary school.

Our imaginary concert is at seven o'clock two nights from now. First, do you take the children? No. Who can babysit them? What time should the sitter come? Should she feed the children? If so, what? What time do you need to start getting ready for your departure? And on and on and on. Now think about a wedding or other celebration and consider the vast amount of planning that goes into an event of that magnitude: the invitations, the venue, the church, the minister, the flowers, the dress, the bridesmaids, the rings, the reception, the food, the cake, the honeymoon.

Most of us are actually quite adept at planning, considering we've been doing it our whole lives. Why, then, can't we see the need to plan most of our meals?

Once I had traveled up the weight-gain road a ways, I saw no way out. It didn't seem possible to lose more than 100 pounds—even with a plan. No matter how many weight-loss programs I tried, I never believed in the importance of meal planning. If I didn't immediately see results with a weight-loss program, then obviously that program wasn't any good, I thought. So I'd quit. I wanted to lose 10 pounds fast, and if I did not lose quickly, I'd stop participating in the program and move onto the next. I never took the time or accepted the responsibility to plan for myself. Instead, I relied on the program's methods and suggestions as the only way to lose weight. When unexpected events came up or daily meals needed cooking, I shut down. I knew what I should be eating, but I never thought that planning would make a difference. I see now that I was destined to fail, for without planning, nothing would have gotten me thin.

When I share my lack of responsibility with other people, they sometimes comment, "You probably just weren't mentally ready to lose weight." I have a small problem with that concept: It is just another excuse, not a reason. Weight loss is not only a mental problem; it is both a physical and an emotional problem. As I said before, if you eat less than your body needs, you lose weight. Conversely, if you eat more than your body needs, you gain weight. The mental aspect does play an enormous role, but it's not the actual physical reason we struggle with our weight. I was overweight because I ate too much. I plodded merrily along from day to day, from year to year, without the slightest plan for turning my weight problem around. I just kept wishing things would magically change.

Your Turn

Do you have a definite plan for weight loss?............................. Yes ❑ No ❑

Can you take responsibility for your own weight issues? .... Yes ❑ No ❑

What is the first step you need to take when making a weight-loss plan?

_____

_____

Fail to Plan, Plan to Fail

As I look back, there were many times during those obese years when I could have stopped my weight problem in its tracks. The one time I did lose a small amount of weight on Weight Watchers, I quit before I even came close to my goal. I quit because I couldn't see the light at the end of the tunnel soon enough. I saw my weight-loss goals as too big for success. I had no long-term plan for achieving my goal by breaking it up into smaller, manageable pieces.

Another time, before I became seriously obese, John and I purchased a piece of exercise equipment called a glider. It was a cross between an exercise bike and a weight machine. I used it and saw some encouraging results but again quit before I really gave myself a chance to get started. After I stopped using it, the glider became a very expensive clothes hanger.

Do you know the saying "Fail to plan, plan to fail"? It applies to weight loss. I didn't fully understand how to develop a healthy eating plan that would result in real, long-term weight loss. I knew dieting, I knew cutting calories to a ridiculous level, and I knew from experience that neither of those approaches work. Although I hated being overweight and hated the way it made me feel, I just couldn't see the forest for the trees. I knew I was fat, but I couldn't understand that my utter failure at establishing and following a plan was making it impossible to get control of my weight.

I want to teach you how to plan your weight loss and to own your plan. Once you take ownership of your plan, it will be easier to lose weight and keep it off. When you think about it, the Fit to the Finish plan is easy. The three points—fat percentage, portion control, and exercise—are simple to understand and simple to follow. What's not so simple is that as the weeks and months roll by, you will be constantly confronted by different situations, holidays, and stressors. You will need to fine-tune your weight-loss plan to accommodate those varying life circumstances.

From the beginning, I knew that limiting my fat intake to 30 percent of my total calories required some planning. I needed to plan for family meals, personal breakfasts, and lunch with the kids. Healthy snacks had to be on hand, and I knew I couldn't rely on a program to do all that for me. Previously, I had rebelled against the whole idea of developing an eating plan. After all, food was everywhere. It was easy to find. Why plan what you are going to eat when you can just roll through your friendly drive-through restaurant for a meal or snack?

Fortunately, I realized that what I had been doing wasn't working. I decided to try planning meals. Even if you are a free spirit who feels like fighting this concept tooth and nail, give it a try. You may be surprised how much more freedom you feel when you are not running around frantically trying to get a meal together at the last minute. I can't stress enough how freeing having a plan really is.

Your Turn

How often do you plan breakfast, lunch, dinner, and snacks? _____
_____
_____

What is the outcome of your planning efforts? _____
_____
_____

Do you see benefits to planning specific meals?...................... Yes ❑ No ❑
_____
_____

List the five home-prepared meals you make most often: _____
_____
_____
_____

What did you have for dinner last week (including restaurant meals)?

Day 1   _____
Day 2   _____
Day 3   _____
Day 4   _____
Day 5   _____
Day 6   _____
Day 7   _____

Did you know when the week started what you
would have for dinner each day?.. Yes ❑ No ❑

Why or why not?
_____
_____

Have you ever planned meals before? .... Yes ❑ No ❑

How comfortable do you feel with making recipe substitutions—for example, subbing yogurt for sour cream or fat-free for full-fat products?

_____

_____

_____

How could your family's favorite meals be prepared in a more healthy way? _____

_____

_____

Your answers will reveal whether you are a planner. If you are, this next section will be fun for you. If you are not, you will have to work a little harder.

Grocery Store Planning

I am an expert grocery shopper. I couldn't always claim that title, but the longer I have maintained my weight, the better I've gotten at shopping. Not only can I spot a bargain, but I have also learned how to use grocery store sales circulars to plan nutritious meals on a budget. This saves me money. It also sets me apart from the 70 percent of Americans who at 4:00 p.m. on any given day don't know what they are having for dinner. You can become an expert grocery shopper too. Start with the three steps below.

Step 1: Plan Your Meals and Snacks for the Week
Use the meal planning worksheet in appendix G to plan your meals for the week. Grocery store circulars can help you plan less-expensive meals.

As you plan your meals, look for ways to substitute out high-fat and high-calorie items. For examples, see ten healthy eating tips in appendix H. Consider not only the main meals of the day but also snacks and sweets. For examples, see healthy meal and snack ideas in appendix I.

Step 2: Make a Grocery List
I know it's a pain to sit down and make that list, but if you don't plan what you are going to buy, you are obviously not planning what you are going

to eat for the week. Refer to your meal plan and use the grocery list template in appendix J to get started.

Step 3: Go Shopping

Grab your coupons, your list, and a good, positive attitude and head to your favorite grocery store. Always start shopping on the perimeter and buy as little processed food as possible.

Avoiding Temptation at the Grocery Story

Once I got started, I found planning the three main meals of the day easy. Where I ran into problems was trying to plan for snacks. What snacks could I have in the house that I would not be tempted to consume in one sitting? At the store, I'd start out with the best intentions, but it was very tempting to purchase my trigger foods and use the children as an excuse. "Well," I'd reason, "Rachel is doing so well in school, and she really enjoys these chocolate chip cookies, so I'll just buy a pack for her." It took great willpower to resist buying those cookies. I eventually made a list of snacks and treats I could and couldn't have around the house. This list reminded me what I should and shouldn't buy. Included on the list of treats I could have around the house were coconut cookies, which I didn't like but the children did. Not included were Oreo cookies.

When you are grocery shopping, bypass your trigger foods. If an errant chocolate item mysteriously makes its way into your basket, take it

Getting Noticed

As I started losing weight, even the cashiers in the grocery store noticed the change in my appearance. After the first 50 pounds, when people were just beginning to see the difference, cashiers would remark, "Wow, you have lost weight." As the weight continued to come off, the comments got more enthusiastic and the questions more pointed. One of the cashiers even ended up attending my Fit to the Finish class.

out. If you take children shopping with you, establish some ground rules before going in. My children quickly understood that I was not going to buy junk food on a regular basis anymore, and they were okay with that. They didn't miss the junk, because I made sure we had lots of healthier choices. I made celery interesting by filling the stalks with peanut butter and raisins. I let the kids mash chickpeas to make hummus for carrot sticks. I used raisins to make faces on their whole-wheat toast. Occasionally, I would let them pick out a piece of candy at the checkout counter, but the days of buying a pound of M&M's for me to eat by myself were gone for good.

Instead of filling my cart with junky, high-fat, processed food, I left the grocery store with a cart full of fresh fruit, healthy vegetables, wholegrain breads, raisins, nuts, popcorn, yogurt, milk, reduced-fat cheese, baked chips and pretzels, and dried beans.

When you have returned from the store and unpacked all your healthy food choices, step back and give yourself a pat on the back. You may even find that you spent less money because you didn't buy as many processed foods. However, healthy whole foods can require additional preparation. And if you work outside the home, it's difficult to walk in the door at 5:30 and start making an entire meal from scratch. So prepare as much of your meals ahead of time as you can. If you can do things to make meal prep easier, do them. Here are some tips.

Food Preparation Tips

Cooking meat is often the most time-consuming part of meal prep. To minimize it, buy chicken breasts on sale. Either roast or boil the chicken until it's thoroughly done. Shred the chicken, store it in 2-cup portions, and freeze it. When properly wrapped, frozen chicken is good for several months. It's great for casseroles, chicken salad, fajitas, tacos, and soups. You can come home, put the frozen chicken in your microwave, and hit the defrost setting. If you do not like using microwave ovens, put the frozen chicken in your refrigerator first thing in the morning, so it will be thawed and ready to use when you are ready to prepare dinner.

If lean ground beef or turkey is on sale, buy several pounds. Brown the meat, rinse it off (this gets rid of some fat calories), and freeze it in

1-cup serving sizes. You can use it in any dish that requires ground beef or turkey, such as tacos, lasagna, wraps, soups, and chili.

I chop five or six onions and green peppers at a time and put them in freezer bags, for later use in soups and casseroles. I do the same thing with carrots, corn on the cob, asparagus, broccoli, peas, and tomatoes.

Using low-fat cheese in a recipe? It is often less expensive to grate your own cheese than to buy it already grated. Grate the amount of cheese you need for the week and store it in plastic bags. Most hard cheeses freeze for up to six months.

Is rice part of your weekly menu? Rice freezes beautifully. Make a double batch, use what you need that night, and freeze the rest. Thaw it in the refrigerator or on the defrost setting of your microwave. No one will ever know it had been frozen.

Crock-Pot meals are a good alternative to eating out. I love coming home after a day out to the smell of dinner cooking. Several low-fat cookbooks are specifically geared for Crock-Pot cooking. One I particularly like is *Slow Cooker* from *Cooking Light* magazine.

I've found that a little preparation goes a long way toward making nightly meals easier and more pleasant. If 50 percent of your meal is ready when you get home, you will be far less tempted to swing through a fast-food restaurant. If you are out all day running errands, knowing you have cooked chicken and chopped vegetables in the freezer will take away the strong temptation to run by the pizza parlor. Many times, my preplanning has kept money in our wallets and kept fat from our hips.

Your Turn

What other foods can be prepared ahead of time? _____
_____
_____
_____
_____
_____

Are you willing to do some preprep work? .... Yes ❑ No ❑

Can family members help with this work? .... Yes ❑ No ❑

What are the benefits of having some food prep done before you get home or at the end of a busy day with the children? _____

_____

_____

_____

_____

When You Stumble

Now that you've planned, made lists, shopped, and preprepped, all you have to do is follow your plan. Don't you love it when I say, "All you have to do"? That's where it gets hard sometimes. Food is such an important part of daily life, and for some people it is a friend who never quits. If you have emotional attachments to food, it can be hard to stick to a meal plan. Even though you know you have a healthy lunch in the break room refrigerator, or all the good ingredients to make a satisfying lunch at home, it's still easy to abandon your good intentions and eat something else instead, or to eat food in addition to what you have planned. This will happen to you, so remember to just start over right away. Go back to eating what you had planned for the next meal, knowing that you have the tools, knowledge, and confidence to get back on track and stay on track.

As you begin seriously planning your meals, you may be surprised to find, as I did, that you are less hungry than you anticipated. You may find that because you are filling up on quality foods, you are more satisfied throughout the day. I found I was more physically satisfied and more emotionally satisfied as well. Each time the choices I made were positive, it gave me a little bit more confidence that I could succeed. I could make good choices, and I could lose weight.

Handling Celebrations in Healthy Style

Everyday meal and snack planning becomes second nature after a few weeks of practice. Like anything else in our lives, once we work at something, we become proficient. Holidays and special occasions can throw a monkey wrench into good intentions and the best laid plans, however. During the ten years I was obese, we had hundreds of celebrations, including birthdays, anniversaries, Christmases, and children's birthdays. We also participated in numerous celebrations and special occasions with friends and relatives. As a perpetual dieter, I spent more time thinking of ways to cheat than thinking of ways to succeed. Every single holiday that rolled around on the calendar was another perfect reason to take a break from my diet.

The year was 1994, and I was once again trying to lose weight. That year, when I finally got concerned enough to again join Weight Watchers, I had the best of intentions. Of course, I was going to lose weight this time. I tried semihard for the first week and saw a loss of 1 pound. That was good, especially since I'd cheated a little bit. The second week was okay, but during the third week, a holiday rolled around. It was Father's Day.

Father's Day was John's day, and I wanted to make it special for him. Even though Father's Day was on a Sunday, I decided that it would be awfully nice to make him his favorite desserts all week long. So beginning on the Monday before Father's Day, I started cooking. Monday: chocolate cookies; Tuesday: seven-layer bars; Wednesday: ice cream with crushed Oreos . . . you get the picture. Did John request all that food? No. I wanted all that food and used the upcoming holiday to justify my choices. Each day of Father's Day week, I woke up and thought about the upcoming dessert that night. I forced myself to wait until late afternoon to make the dessert, so I wouldn't be tempted to eat the whole thing myself, which had happened before. After dinner we all enjoyed John's special dessert. By the time Father's Day Sunday came around, the whole family was a little bit burned out on dessert, but we rallied to eat yet another cake. While reading that paragraph, did you forget, as I did, that I was dieting that week? I was supposed to be watching what I ate and trying to lose weight. What happened to my good intentions? A holiday—also known as the best excuse in the book.

I was also guilty of using the time between Halloween and New Year's as a big eating fest. The appearance of Halloween candy in stores started my food extravaganza, and I loved every minute of it. Diet or not, I was going to enjoy the holiday season. But I didn't just enjoy the individual meals for each holiday. I enjoyed all the meals of the holiday months. Time after time, I used the holiday season as an excuse to quit my plan.

Most of us have heard people complain about the commercialization of certain holidays and the fact that children are spoiled with holiday presents and goodies. I never bothered with those debates, because the more goodies I had around at holidays, the happier I was. Christmas is a wonderful holiday, not just because of the meaning behind it but also because of the food that comes with it—especially the candy.

I was always happy when Halloween candy disappeared off store shelves, knowing it would be replaced by Christmas candy. I'd start buying Christmas candy early in November, when it was on sale. My plan was to buy it in increments to save money. But the red-and-green foil packages begged to be opened, and the candy bags usually didn't even make it home from the grocery store in one piece. I'd rip a bag open and tell myself, *I'm only going to eat two.* Crunch, crunch. *Okay, just one more.* After repeating this process over and over during the ten-minute drive home, I'd realize with consternation that half the bag was gone. I'd stuff the bag in my purse, nonchalantly walk in the house, and help the family unload the groceries. The first chance I got, I'd hide the half-empty bag in my dresser drawer to be enjoyed at a later time.

I repeated this fruitless "money-saving" effort time and time again throughout November and December. When Christmas came close, I'd innocently ask John, "Do you think we should go ahead and get some candy for stockings?" He'd agree, and off we'd go to buy more. I loved Christmas!

Holidays come all the time. Special occasions will always occur. Our lives are usually enriched and fulfilled by celebrations with family, friends, and coworkers. Because these special times won't stop for your weight-loss efforts, you must develop a strategy to deal with the food that inevitably surrounds the holiday at hand.

Your Turn

Have you ever tried to lose weight when a holiday
celebration was coming up?... Yes ❑ No ❑

What were the circumstances? _____

_____

_____

_____

Were you successful? .... Yes ❑ No ❑

Did you continue with your diet after the holiday? .... Yes ❑ No ❑

Is Food the Point?

Conquering the holiday season without gaining weight requires you to
keep your commitment to changing your eating habits and exercising
regularly. If you just shrug your shoulders and say you are going to do
your best, you'll never make it through. And once you have fallen off the
weight-loss wagon, it can be extremely difficult to get back on. Let's think
about the purpose of holidays. They are for remembrance, appreciation,
celebration, acknowledgment, and contemplation. Holidays are important parts of our lives and should be celebrated with much excitement
and ceremony.

In our family, we celebrate everything from the first day of spring
to getting an A in algebra, but we no longer put all the emphasis on
food. When I finally lost weight and began the process of learning to
maintain the loss, I realized that holidays aren't only about the food
but about the people you are with. Spending time with the family
you love is reward enough; food is secondary. Easy? No. It's not easy
to readjust your thinking in that way. So programmed are we to surround our holidays with food that we sometimes overlook the real
reason for gathering.

Why use wonderful celebrations as an excuse for eating anything and
everything we want? Perhaps for the same reason we eat too much when

we eat out. We look at holidays as a time to treat ourselves. Holidays also call for special menu items, such as the Jewish tradition of serving latkes, or potato pancakes during Hanukkah. Whatever your cultural background, you can enjoy the traditions and celebrate your heritage without overeating.

Your Turn

What is your favorite holiday? _____

_____

_____

_____

Why? _____

_____

_____

_____

_____

Is it hard for you to control your food intake on that
holiday?... Yes ❑ No ❑

What foods associated with that holiday do you enjoy? _____

_____

_____

_____

_____

Do you ever feel that you lose sight of what you
are celebrating?... Yes ❑ No ❑

Focus on the Holiday

We learned in an earlier chapter to focus on restaurant meals as just meals, not treats. Let's think of holiday meals in a similar manner.

Appreciate the Holiday for the Holiday's Sake
In our family, birthdays are huge. If it is your birthday, you are pampered and get all kinds of extra attention. You get out of some chores
and get to pick your favorite meals and dessert. With all the yummy
food around, it is easy to lose sight of the person we are honoring. I was
thankful that John loved seven-layer cookie bars, and I happily made
and ate them. I was ecstatic that he wanted that fabulous three-layer
chocolate cake for his birthday, and I couldn't wait to eat it. His actual
birthday party was almost a letdown, because all the focus was on food
and not on him.

Avoid Using Holidays as a Free-for-All Eating Fest
Remember that holidays are for celebrating events, not solely for eating. It's
too easy to justify eating candy or baking special seasonal desserts under
the guise of the holiday celebration. The weeks leading up to Christmas
in my family are often full of kid's school activities, such as concerts and
cantatas, end-of-semester programs, and final exams. If you do not have
children, you will still be invited to seasonal parties, concerts, work celebrations, and family gatherings. I was frequently asked to make treats
for end-of-the season events and would gladly do so. After all, this was a
legitimate reason to bake. I would bake enough to take—and enough to
eat myself. I used the holiday as an excuse to fuel my overeating problem.

Enjoy Yourself within Reason
I'm not saying that you can't have Grandma Jane's famous fruitcake, Aunt
Delores's custard pie, or Uncle Ben's brownies. I am saying that you must
carefully choose what foods you will eat and what foods you will say "no
thank-you" to. If you can't learn to say those two words, you will be one
of the millions of Americans who gain an average of 7 pounds during the
months of November and December. If you don't lose the weight gained
after the holidays, you will put on pound after pound, year after year.

When holiday parties come around and the buffet lines are long and
welcoming, you can employ some specific strategies to stay on track.

Set limits: Set mental limits as to what you will and will not eat for
any given occasion. Most of us have a general idea what kind of food will
be served at an event. At a birthday party, I allow myself a small piece of
cake (if I like the flavor) or a small scoop of ice cream, but not both. At a

wedding or other large party, I have the fruits and veggies but pass on the big gooey desserts.

Have a small snack before you leave the house: This will help fill you up, so when your eyes are tickled by the smorgasbord of goodies, your stomach will tell your brain, "I'm already full." Then you can choose wisely from the available offerings.

Drink water on the way: Drink water on the way there, so that when you arrive, your stomach isn't empty. This trick will help cut down on the amount of food you consume.

Don't allow others to make you feel guilty: I can't tell you how many times at celebrations, friends encouraged me to eat "just one piece" because it was a holiday. I politely refused but was often surprised by my friends' lack of sensitivity to my desire to get and stay healthy. I had to reach the point where my decision to stay healthy was more important than eating what a friend wanted me to eat. This wasn't always easy, but as long as I was polite, I knew I had made a good decision for myself.

Just remember, you will be the one who later suffers the emotional and physical consequences that follow poor choices at holiday gatherings. If you plan carefully and stay mindful of what you're putting in your mouth, you can be one of the few who loses or maintains weight over the major holiday season.

Planning makes our lives easier. Pick one aspect of this chapter to work on at a time. You might be able to plan dinners but have to work toward lunch planning. That's okay. By tackling each category separately, you will see your success level steadily increase. Holidays and special occasions bring joy to us. Celebrate with abandon, but plan carefully.

17

Moving into Maintenance

This can be the last time you lose weight. Wow. When you see it in writing, what does that mean for you? You can do it this last time and never have to go through the pain, emotional trauma, and hard work to lose weight again.

When I lost 150 pounds, I didn't regain my weight for one simple reason: I didn't stop utilizing the tools and techniques I used when losing weight. I designed the Fit to the Finish plan to be a plan for life, not a short-term diet. If you lose weight by following the three points of the plan, and continue following those guidelines in the years to come, you should be able to maintain your weight loss as I have.

You are on your way to becoming the size you desire. As you move toward that goal, take some time to do a few things along the way.

Get Rid of the Fat Clothes

Get rid of clothes that no longer fit. As you lose weight, your clothes will start to become too big for you. Don't keep them. Donate them to charity or have a garage sale. It's a great feeling to know you will never wear that pair of "fat pants" again.

Speaking of fat pants, I'll share one more embarrassing moment. One hot Saturday, we decided to hold a yard sale. We were doing a brisk business. After all, fifty cents per clothing item is a pretty good deal. About midway through the morning, a car pulled up and a very large woman got out, along with some of her friends. They looked around at our stuff, one of the ladies bought a household item or two, and they prepared to leave. Before they left the sale, the extremely large lady came up to me and said, "Are you selling any of your sized clothes?"

I looked at her and said, "Excuse me?"

She said again, "Are you selling your clothes?"

I said, "No—sorry." She left with her friends, and I was left staring in disbelief. I hoofed over to John and asked him a question I would immediately regret. I said, "Am I as big as that woman walking away over there?"

He shrugged as if to say, "I'm not sure."

"Am I?" I demanded to know.

He finally said, "Well, actually you are a little bigger than she is. Why?" I told him why and immediately fell into a depression that lasted the rest of the day, eased only by the handfuls of chocolate I ate to make up for the hurt.

As I lost weight, I gladly sold or gave away my clothes to ladies who really were bigger than I was. I kept one T-shirt (pictured below), one dress, and one maternity shirt as a memento of where I had been and

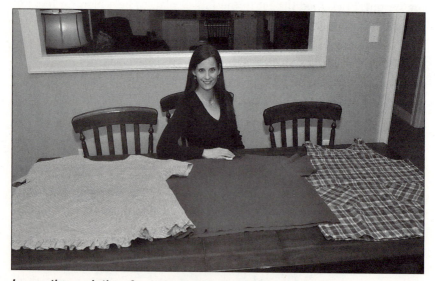

I wore these clothes for many years and hated putting them on. These are the only three items of fat clothing that I kept.

where I never wanted to be again. I encourage you to do the same. Keep one big pair of pants or shirt, but get rid of the rest. If you don't discard your big clothes as you lose weight, you will always know they are in your closet—just in case. Let's not have a "just in case" wardrobe this time.

Avoiding the Weight-Loss/Weight-Gain Cycle

If you've been on other diet plans, you have probably experienced the weight-loss/weight-gain cycle. Once I lost 150 pounds, I really didn't want to gain it back. I was truly serious about maintaining my weight loss and not having to repurchase big-girl clothes or relive the fat life. As I got closer and closer to my goal weight, I began evaluating what I needed to do next. What would make this time different?

To make this time different for you, do the same thing I did. By continuing to follow the plan after you reach your goal, you can maintain your weight. Continuing to follow the plan shouldn't be hard, because you've already changed your habits. Your eating patterns after you reach your goal weight shouldn't be significantly different than when you are in the midst of losing weight.

I remember John asking me as I lost weight, "Won't you be so happy when you can go back to eating Breyer's ice cream and Oreo cookies?" I looked at him and said, "I'm not going back."

"You mean you aren't ever going to have a treat?" he asked.

I told him that of course I was going to have treats on occasion, but I would never again overindulge in food as a salve for emotional discomfort, boredom, or stress. I also told him I was going to follow my plan and plan my food choices accordingly—for life.

You see, there really is no going back. If you go back, you gain back. If you revert to your old eating habits, you will gain back the weight you have lost. Don't do it. We all fight emotional battles when it comes to food. We fight demons from our past. We fight feelings that make us want to flee to food. Ultimately, though, it's within your hands to win those battles. For me, that's where prayer and study come in. When I was losing weight, there weren't too many days when I didn't cry out to God for help. Besides prayer, and a commitment to making good choices, you may be wondering what other strategies I employed to keep my weight where I wanted it to be.

The 3-Pound Limit

Once I reached my goal weight, I continued watching my portion sizes, monitoring the percentage of fat I was consuming, and exercising. I have been through dozens of holidays, birthdays, and celebrations without gaining weight. I have been through stressful times and happy times, busy times and lazy times, all without gaining weight. How?

The first thing I did was give myself a 3-pound limit. Weighing myself every day kept me honest. If I saw the scale creep up 3 pounds, I cut back on snacking, exercised a little harder, and watched what I was eating. It worked, and it was easy because those 2 or 3 pounds fell right off. It's a lot easier to lose 2 or 3 pounds than 10 or 20.

A friend of mine serves as a good example of the benefits of the 3-pound rule. As I was losing weight, she got motivated to lose the 20 pounds she had been carrying around. She asked me what I did and started following the same plan. She lost her 20 pounds within a few months and was ecstatic. But guess what? She didn't follow the 3-pound rule and allowed herself to gain back 5 pounds, then 2 more, and before she knew it she had gained back 10 pounds. She was so annoyed at herself and had to work hard for several long weeks to lose the 10 pounds again. She committed to not letting her weight creep up again. The last time I saw her, ten years later, she was still slim and trim.

Her experience shows why it is important to set an upper weight limit for yourself. Even if you regain weight slowly, over the course of several years, it all adds up. Imagine if I had let my weight creep up 5 to 7 pounds per year over the last dozen years. Now, instead of claiming a 150-pound weight loss, I would have to say that I had lost 150 pounds and gained 84 pounds. Every little pound adds up, especially year by year. Five pounds may not make much of a difference in how your clothes fit, but after ten years, 50 pounds will.

Accountability Partner

The second strategy I suggest for weight maintenance is to have an accountability partner with whom you share your weight gain or loss. I used my husband as an accountability partner, although I did not share the actual number on the scale. I would tell him that I was within my weight range or whether I had gained more than a few pounds. He never made me feel bad for gaining a few pounds. Rather, he told me that I had done such a good job maintaining my weight loss and that he knew I would get my weight back within my goal range.

If you can, find someone with whom you can share your weight struggles and triumphs. Even if you aren't comfortable sharing your actual weight, you might be able to confess that you have allowed your weight to creep up a bit. Sometimes, just knowing you have to share your progress with a friend or spouse helps you get back on track.

Rate Your Food

In my past fat life, I was not discriminating when it came to food. If it looked like food, smelled like food, and tasted like food, I ate it. I didn't really care whether I even liked it.

So the third strategy I suggest—one I still use—is to rate your food. When faced with a tempting food choice, I rate the enjoyment I will get from that food against the enjoyment I experience at my current weight. Quite frankly, that special food has to be pretty good for me to eat it. These days, I definitely have the occasional cookie or bowl of ice cream, but on a daily basis I still watch the amount of sweets I consume. When we eat dinner at friends' houses, I try to be objective about my food choices. I set aside the fact that a friend made food for us and look at my feelings about the food. Is it a dessert I totally love and will be sad if I don't try, or can I pass it up? My goal is to never lose sight of the satisfaction I feel with my current weight and to always keep in mind my desire for lifetime weight maintenance.

One night we were at my grandmother's house. She made a delicious dinner, and I had eaten very well. After dinner, she asked if I wanted some decaf coffee with dessert. I told her I definitely wanted coffee, but I wanted to think about dessert. She said, "Okay, but here's what I have." She put a box of Godiva chocolates on the table and left to start the coffee. I leaned forward and looked into the box. Yum. I thought about my closet full of size-6 dresses. I thought about the chocolates. Was this food good enough for me to eat? Yes it was. I picked one piece and enjoyed it thoroughly—guilt-free—because I had made the decision with care—stopping, evaluating, and waiting.

On the other hand, when a friend had us over for dinner one night, she made a fruit cobbler for dessert. Cobbler was a dessert I could do without. After dinner, I politely declined dessert, knowing that on a scale of 1 to 10, the cobbler was about a 4. I certainly didn't need it. And in evaluating my desire, I really didn't want it. Later, I was very proud of the choice I had made. It was another victory for me, resisting a dessert that previously I would have indulged in. I remember John looking at me saying, "You're not going to try the cobbler?" I told him, "No, I'm full." Later that night, after we returned home, I shared with him my thought process, and he agreed that it certainly seemed to work. I employ this strategy frequently, as mentally rating my food helps me make good choices.

How I Think of Food

I look at food differently now. The year it took me to lose weight was long enough to change my habits and thoughts related to food. People who lose weight using liquid diets or boxed food diets never learn to eat real food during their time of weight loss. That's what makes Fit to the Finish different than other plans. You haven't been eating boxed foods. You haven't been just drinking breakfast and lunch. Most importantly, you haven't been cooking differently for yourself than you do for your family. You haven't even had to count anything.

Holidays and parties used to be all about the food for me. I now look forward to simply celebrating the occasion. I find focusing on the happiness of the person we are honoring to be so much more satisfying than focusing on the food I will be serving. Birthdays and holidays are still special in our families. In fact, in some ways they are more special now, since I really make the effort to communicate my love and appreciation for my family other than just with food.

Food is an important part of my life, as it is yours. But it's not my whole life. I enjoy eating foods of all kinds. I now like to cook, and I find great pleasure in trying new, healthy recipes that I never would have tried in my fat days. I still enjoy baking and presenting my family with special meals. But I no longer think of food as the friend who will never leave me.

I have finally put food in proper perspective, and that took some practice. There were times, after I lost weight, when I found myself thinking about food all day long. I would give myself a little pep talk, find something to keep me busy, and banish the excess thoughts. After a time, I noticed that my obsession with food lessened.

Your Turn

Complete these sentences:

Food is my _____

_____

I want food to be my _____

_____

_____

The Benefits of Being Healthy and Fit

There are so many benefits to being at a healthy weight and to achieving an appropriate level of fitness that I never could list them all here. But following are the ten most commonly cited benefits:

1. Increased energy level
2. Lower cholesterol levels
3. Reduced blood pressure
4. Reduced aches and pains
5. Improved mobility
6. Improved breathing
7. Better sleep
8. Prevention of angina (chest pain caused by decreased oxygen to the heart)
9. Decreased risk of sudden death from heart disease or stroke
10. Prevention or reversal of type 2 diabetes and improved blood sugar levels

And if those health-related benefits aren't enough to convince you to continue on your journey, how about the added benefit of looking better?

Appearance

Being a smaller size and looking better is one obvious benefit of weight loss and maintenance for me. Food became less important than being happy with my appearance. That alone was a very good reason not to overeat. We all want to feel good about ourselves, and part of that good feeling is related to how we look. If you think you look good, you often feel better about yourself. Right or wrong, that is how a lot of us feel. In teaching classes throughout the years, I have heard this sentiment expressed time and time again: "I will just be happier with myself if I can lose this 10 pounds." As my students achieve success and share their stories with me, I see their faces blossom with excitement.

I can't tell you how good it felt when I was finally the size I wanted to be. It's so nice to go into a store, pull clothing off the rack, put it on, and have it fit. Gone are the days when I would close my eyes as I pulled up a pair of pants, hoping against hope that they would actually fit over my thighs. And hoping that if I could get them over my thighs, I would even like the way they looked. I don't feel like a different person when I wear smaller clothes, but I do feel different about myself, and that's very special.

Self-Esteem

When I weigh what I want to weigh, I behave differently as well. Gone are the days of not being able to look certain people in the eye. Thin people often intimidated me. Call it a character flaw if you will, but that's how I felt. When I say that I behave differently now, I'm not saying that I pretend to be someone I'm not. I just feel more confident and sure of myself at a healthy weight.

I no longer hide behind big glasses and ugly clothes, hoping no one will notice me. I feel freer to express my opinions and offer suggestions. As my weight ballooned, I receded into the shadows. I convinced myself that people didn't want to know anything about me. After all, who likes a fat girl? I really didn't need more than two friends, did I? And, to be honest, I felt like those two friends were doing me a favor by being nice to the fat girl. Now I understand that those perceptions were all in my mind, but that doesn't invalidate the way I felt. These days, I realize that people are my friends because they want to be, not out of the desire to do me a favor or because they feel sorry for me.

I can walk into a room and not wonder what people are thinking about me. I operate with increased self-confidence and am more aware of others and their needs. The focus isn't on what people are thinking about me but rather on what I can do for other people. I'm more willing to take the initiative with strangers rather than waiting for people to come to me. I make friends more easily and get to know people faster than I did in the past.

Here's a little story to illustrate this point. As a fat person, I felt judged. I was ridiculed. I endured humiliation. At 300 pounds, physical activity was difficult for me. Once I started losing a substantial amount of weight, the positive comments were encouraging. Sometimes, though, I secretly worried that I would not be able to keep up the weight loss and achieve my goals. I also worried that no matter how much I tried, some people would still perceive me as fat.

One day in November 1997, my family and I went to SeaWorld with my mom. We loaded up the van and drove to Orlando. At this point, I had lost about 110 pounds. What a difference it made. Instead of lumbering through the park with a fake smile pasted on my face, I enthusiastically walked from show to show and exhibit to exhibit. At times it felt as though my family had to hurry to keep up with me instead of vice versa. It was turning out to be a great day.

The highlight of the day came as we sat in the big arena to watch the killer whale show. As we were waiting for the show to begin, we watched the beautiful killer whales swim around the large pool. They were amazing. Imagine my surprise when a SeaWorld employee came up to my family, walked over to *me*, and asked if I'd like to be the trainer's helper for the show. Very calmly I said, "Sure." However, in my mind I was screaming, *me, me?* I knew that if I had weighed 300 pounds, she would *not* have selected me to be the helper. As a Floridian, I had been to amusement parks countless times and had never seen a morbidly obese person asked to assist the trainer.

It was a wonderful experience to have the killer whale trainer point to me and ask me to come down. I walked down the stairs and greeted her. I stood in front of the huge audience, did what she asked, and saw my picture up on the gigantic LCD screen. As I stood there, I wanted to cry and laugh at the same time. I realized that people didn't see me as obese anymore. I realized that I had passed through the fire and come out whole. All the hard work and dedication was paying off, and I was proud. And I felt validated.

I remember looking over at John and the children. The girls were waving and bouncing in their seats, and the smile on John's face was a memory I'll always carry. When my little part in the show was over, I sat back down. John put his arm around me and said, "That was one memory I'll never forget." I leaned into him and said, "Me neither." For the rest of the day, as I walked around the park, people who had been at that show said, "There's the girl who got to pet Shamu." I thought to myself, *Yes, and here's the woman who will never go back to being fat again.*

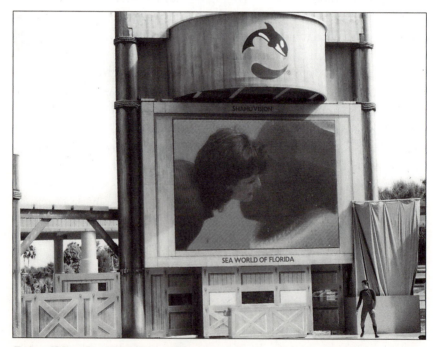

Being "Miss SeaWorld" for that moment was validation that I was no longer the fat, overlooked person that I had been for the previous ten years.

Physical Energy

Once, when I weighed about 275 pounds, I tried to rewallpaper the bathroom in a house we were updating. I attempted to do the project myself and actually finished it. That night I was so exhausted from the physical activity that I went to bed at eight o'clock. The following days found me sitting around eating chocolate, trying to regain my energy. These days, even with a large family, I find the energy to do whatever I want. Paint the living room? Not a problem. Weed the flower beds? Done, and with energy to spare. I no longer have to ration my activities around my energy level. Now my activities are rationed only by the hours in the day.

It goes without saying that I enjoy being more physically active. I exercise six days a week and often run up and down the driveway, trying to help my four-year-old son ride his bike or balance on his scooter. Such times spent with my children are invaluable and unforgettable.

Your Turn

Is there anything you'd like to do that requires more
energy than you have right now?.. Yes ❏ No ❏

How can getting more fit help you achieve your goals?

_____

_____

_____

Things to Avoid

As you get closer to your goal, don't get complacent. Don't revert to your previous eating habits. Keep watching your fat percentage and keep exercising. Don't abandon your support system. If you let down your guard, you could hurt your chances for long-term success. Ask people who have regained weight they had previously lost, and they will all tell you that they let down their guards about healthy eating. I've said all along that I want you to quit dieting and start living. Hopefully, as you've

Family Matters

The personal benefits to losing 150 pounds were immediately obvious to anyone who saw me, or looked at before pictures of me. I looked better, I could move around more easily, and I was undoubtedly healthier. A side benefit that may be just as important was the impact that my weight loss had on my family. When I began losing weight, my children were young enough that I could easily influence and control their food intake. However, I often think about what would have happened to them if I had not lost weight and changed our eating habits.

Would my children have ended up being overweight or obese like the majority of American children are today? Probably. Why wouldn't they have been? After all, I was feeding them a diet too high in processed foods, allowing them to eat fast food several nights a week, and keeping all sorts of candy and cookies in the house. As they grew up, my inability to eat a healthy diet would have likely influenced their choices. After all, if Mom eats brownies for breakfast, why can't they?

Over the years since I've lost weight, I see firsthand the benefits of healthy living in my kids. We have lively discussions at the dinner table about eating healthy foods, what types of food additives manufacturers put in foods, and how to enjoy the occasional treat without feeling guilty. Each of them understands that although no food is strictly off limits, certain foods such as chips, candy, or ice cream should be enjoyed in moderation.

My fifth and sixth children, aged eight and six, enjoy looking at the sides of cereal boxes or yogurt containers and deciding whose yogurt or cereal is healthier. My teenaged children choose not to drink sodas or sweetened drinks because "water is best." Even my husband watches his fat, sodium, and sugar intake.

The children enjoy being active, love cooking with me, and often thank me for making sure they understand what a healthy diet looks like. I am forever grateful that I got myself out of the obesity trap and didn't drag my family down there with me.

journeyed through this book, you have gotten out of the dieting mindset and into the healthy living and eating mindset.

When you reach your goal weight, it is very easy to become complacent. Complacency is dangerous. When I got complacent, I gained weight back very quickly. I thought, "I'm where I want to be, so let's go get some ice cream!" Wrong. If you think like that, you will gain your weight back. Becoming fit takes a lot of focused thought and practice. Once you are there, you must still focus on making the right choices. The longer you practice making good choices, the more natural it becomes. Before long, you won't need to think about it so much.

Reaching my goal wasn't the end. I found that the months following my weight loss were actually more difficult than the last few months of losing weight. It was a battle to stay on top of my eating habits and to figure out the right balance between eating enough to maintain my weight and not eating so much as to gain weight. It took a little bit of time to get it right, but once I did, weight maintenance was easy.

If you revert to your previous eating habits and stop watching the fat percentage in foods, you know what will happen. The weight you worked so hard to lose will come back. Before you know it, you will see the scale creep back up and your pants become tight. Once you reach your goal, you can have the occasional treat, but you can't have treats all the time or you will regain weight. The longer you are at your goal weight, the easier it will be to make the right choices.

I encourage you to think of weight loss as a process, not a period of time. The process includes getting started, journeying through choices, achieving success, and maintaining your weight. If you work through each process honestly and with diligence, you can have lifetime success. It's in your hands.

Exercise is a vital component of weight maintenance. When you are losing weight, exercise helps burn off excess fat and calories. When you are at your goal weight, exercise keeps you fit and lets you have the occasional treat without gaining weight. When I exercise, I can eat more food. I didn't think of exercise in those terms when I was losing weight, because that wasn't the point of exercise. But now that I'm at my goal weight, exercise has the added benefit of allowing me some extra calories each day. Exercise also helps me mentally. With a large family, life can be stressful at times. Exercising gives me a few minutes alone to focus on myself and to set goals for the day.

If you've established a strong support system, don't give up on it now. Once you reach your goal weight, the friends and family who supported you throughout your journey can move to a different role. Now they can encourage you to make the right choices and can keep you honest if you start to fall off the wagon. Thank them for their help and let them know you are not ready to go it alone yet.

Final Words

I want to thank you for reading this book. I hope that each of you has the success that I have had. Losing weight and keeping it off has been a life-changing experience that I wouldn't trade for anything in the world. As difficult as it was to be fat, the rewards of helping people achieve what I achieved outweigh the ten years of pain.

As you go forth on your quest, keep in mind that all things are possible. Don't give up, no matter how hard the road seems. You can be Fit to the Finish!

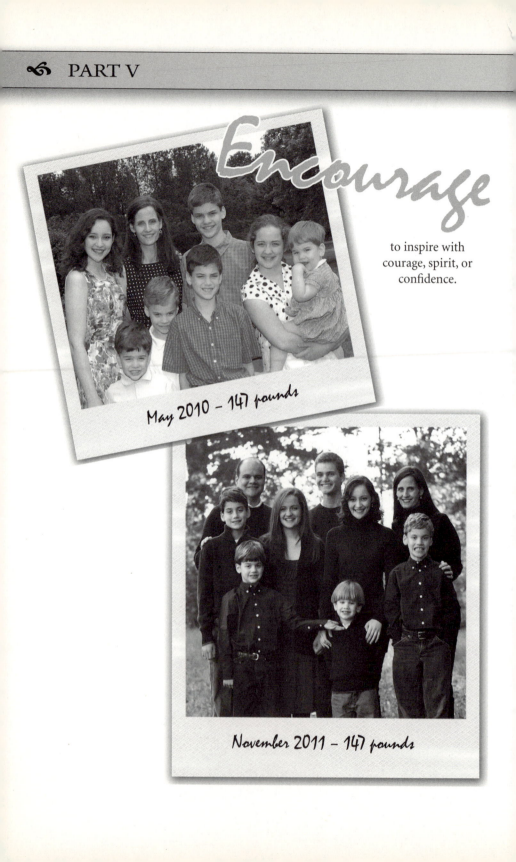

Encourage

to inspire with courage, spirit, or confidence.

May 2010 – 147 pounds

November 2011 – 147 pounds

Recipes

Although a weight-loss book can be complete without recipes, I want to give you some of the recipes that my family and I enjoy. All of them have an appropriate amount of fat and contain healthy, nutritious ingredients. Most of the recipes take little time to prepare.

At the beginning of each recipe, I give you a short description to help you decide whether your family will enjoy the dish.

Bon appétit!

Recipe Index

Recipe Index

Breakfasts to Begin the Day Right

Steel-Cut Oatmeal

Steel-cut oatmeal gives you a nutty flavor that surpasses the taste of ordinary oatmeal. The extra preparation time is worth the effort.

Ingredients
1 c steel-cut oats
3½ c boiling water
1 c skim milk
1 tsp brown sugar
1 tsp cinnamon

Directions
Boil the water in a medium-size saucepan. Slowly pour the oats into the water, stirring constantly. Immediately reduce the temperature to low and allow the oats to simmer for 20 to 25 minutes. Stir occasionally. Warm the milk in the microwave or on the stove. Pour the warmed milk into the steel-cut oats. Stir to combine and allow the mixture to cook for another 10 to 15 minutes, or until the oats are soft enough for your taste. Divide the mixture into two small bowls. Sprinkle with a mixture of brown sugar and cinnamon.

Serves 2

Nutrition Facts
Per serving: 183 Calories (13% from Fat, 20% from Protein, 67% from Carbohydrate); 9 g Protein; 3 g Total Fat; 1 g Saturated Fat, 0.8 g Polyunsaturated Fat; 1 g Monounsaturated Fat; 31 g Carbohydrate; 4 g Fiber; 1 g Sugar; 42 mg Sodium; 1 mg Cholesterol

Whole-Wheat Pancakes

If you are looking for a filling breakfast, grind your own whole wheat as I do or use 100 percent organic whole wheat from your local grocery store.

Ingredients
1 c whole-wheat flour
2 tsp baking powder
1/4 tsp salt
2 tbsp honey
1/2 tbsp canola oil
1 c low-fat buttermilk
2 large eggs

Directions
For the best results, mix the wet and dry ingredients separately. Mix the whole-wheat flour, baking powder, and salt in one bowl. In a separate bowl, mix the honey, oil, buttermilk, and eggs.

Make a well in the dry mixture and slowly pour the wet ingredients into the well. Mix with a spoon until completely combined. Lumps in the batter are okay, as they will break apart in cooking.

Heat up a griddle or frying pan. Spray the pan with cooking spray to prevent the pancakes from sticking. Pour about 1/4 cup batter into different sections of the pan. Allow to cook for 3 to 5 minutes. Turn the pancakes over when the edges are set and the middles are bubbling. Cook for a few more minutes.

Add some blueberries to your pancake batter for added nutrition.

Serves 4

Nutrition Facts
Per Serving: 209 Calories (21% from Fat, 17% from Protein, 62% from Carbohydrate); 9.3 g Protein; 5.2 g Total Fat; 1.3 g Saturated Fat, 1.3 g Polyunsaturated Fat; 2.3 g Monounsaturated Fat; 32.6 g Carbohydrate; 3.7 g Fiber; 11.7 g Sugar; 208 mg Sodium; 95 mg Cholesterol

Egg White Omelets

This cholesterol-free version of a standard omelet will fill you up but with few calories and lots of protein.

Ingredients

3 large egg whites
2 tsp water
1 tsp dill (dried or fresh)
dash of pepper
1 cup finely chopped or
    shredded spinach
1 Roma tomato, diced
1/4 cup reduced-fat cheddar
    cheese

Directions

Whisk the egg whites, water, dill, and pepper together in a small mixing bowl. Mix until the mixture appears set and you can see soft peaks beginni ng to form. Set the other ingredients aside on a plate or bowl.

Spray a small frying pan with nonstick cooking spray. Heat the pan for about 60 seconds. Slowly pour the beaten egg white mixture into your heated pan. Allow the eggs to cook undisturbed until they start to set.

Sprinkle the spinach, tomatoes, and cheese over half the omelet. Fold the half without toppings over the half with toppings. Cook 2 to 4 more minutes. Remove the omelet from the pan and enjoy.

Serves 1

Nutrition Facts

Per Serving: 119 Calories (17% from Fat, 67% from Protein, 16% from Carbohydrate); 20 g Protein; 2.3 g Total Fat; 1.3 g Saturated Fat; .1 g Polyunsaturated Fat; 0.6 g Monounsaturated Fat; 4.5 g Carbohydrate; 1.3 g Fiber; .1 g Sugar; 367 mg Sodium; 5.9 mg Cholesterol

Healthy Breakfast Parfait

For a breakfast that you and your kids will love, make a quick breakfast parfait. It gives you protein, whole grains, and fruit in one easy-to-eat dish.

Ingredients

1 c fat-free or low-fat vanilla
    Greek yogurt
1/2 c fruit, such as chopped
    strawberries, blueberries,
    peaches, or bananas
1/4 c low-fat granola, with no
    raisins

Directions

Spoon 1/2 cup Greek yogurt into the bottom of a parfait cup or drinking glass. Layer 1/4 cup fruit and 1/4 cup granola on top. Carefully spoon the remainder of the Greek yogurt on top of the granola. Repeat layers, finishing with granola.

Serves 2

Nutrition Facts

Per Serving: 138 Calories (5% from Fat, 32% from Protein, 63% from Carbohydrate); 11 g Protein; 0.8 g Total Fat; 0.1 g Saturated Fat; 0.2 g Polyunsaturated Fat; 0.4 g Monounsaturated Fat; 22 g Carbohydrate; 1.8 g Fiber; 13 g Sugar; 74 mg Sodium; 0 mg Cholesterol (Nutrition information based on using strawberries as the fruit.)

Tasty and Simple Vegetable Dishes

Couscous and Vegetables

Couscous is an easy-to-prepare grain that goes well with a variety of vegetables.

Ingredients
1 c water
1 c whole-wheat couscous
1/2 tbsp extra-virgin olive oil
1/2 c finely diced onion
1 clove garlic, finely minced
1/2 c chopped orange or red pepper
1/2 c chopped zucchini
2 tsp no-salt seasoning

Directions
In a small saucepan, heat the water to a rapid boil. Slowly pour the couscous into the boiling water. Stir briefly, cover the pan, and remove from the heat. Heat the olive oil in a small skillet. Add the onion and garlic. Sauté for 1 to 2 minutes. Add the peppers, zucchini, and seasoning. Cook until the vegetables are crisp-tender. Spoon the couscous onto a serving plate. Top with the cooked vegetable mixture and mix gently with a fork.

Serves 4

Nutrition Facts
Per Serving: 77 Calories (21 from Fat, 10% from Protein, 69% from Carbohydrate); 2.1 g Protein; 1.8 g Total Fat; 0.3 g Saturated Fat; 0.2 g Polyunsaturated Fat; 1.3 g Monounsaturated Fat; 13.4 g Carbohydrate; 1.4 g Fiber; 0.4 g Sugar; 3.8 mg Sodium; 0 mg Cholesterol

Roasted Potatoes with Greek Seasoning

These potatoes go with a variety of main dishes, from seafood to beef.
A serving of potatoes is 1/2 cup.

Ingredients
2 medium-size white potatoes
1 tbsp olive oil
1 tbsp lemon or lime juice
1 tbsp sodium-free Greek seasoning

Directions
Preheat oven to 450 degrees. Scrub potatoes under running water. Cut into large bite-sized pieces. Mix the cut potatoes with the oil, lemon or lime juice, and Greek seasoning. Place potatoes on a baking sheet sprayed with nonstick spray. Bake for 30 to 45 minutes or until potatoes are crispy, browned, and tender.

Serves 4

Nutrition Facts
Per Serving: 103 Calories (29% from Fat, 5% from Protein, 66% from Carbohydrate); 1.5 g Protein; 3.5 g Total Fat; 0.5 g Saturated Fat; 0.3 g Polyunsaturated Fat; 2.5 g Monounsaturated Fat; 17.1 g Carbohydrate; 1.2 g Fiber; 0 g Sugar; 4.7 mg Sodium; 0 mg Cholesterol

Spiced Carrots

This is a great alternative to syrupy sweet carrots. These are soft, healthy, and nicely seasoned.

Ingredients
2 c coarsely chopped carrots
1/8 c brown sugar
1 tbsp lemon juice
1 tbsp no-salt seasoning mix
1/4 tsp cumin
1 tbsp paprika
1 c water

Directions
Place all ingredients into a medium-size saucepan. Stir once and bring to a boil. Stir occasionally and cook until the carrots are soft but not falling apart. Add more water if needed.

Serves 4

Nutrition Facts
Per Serving: 45 Calories (0.6% from Fat, 5.3% from Protein, 94% from Carbohydrate); 0.6 g Protein; 0.3 g Total Fat; 0 g Saturated Fat; 0.2 g Polyunsaturated Fat; 0 g Monounsaturated Fat; 10.5 g Carbohydrate; 1.6 g Fiber; 8.8 g Sugar; 26.2 mg Sodium; 0 mg Cholesterol

Quinoa Pilaf

If you've never tried quinoa, do not be afraid to try this dish. It will fill you up and give you a serving of whole grains and vegetables.

Ingredients
3 tbsp chopped shallots
1 c green or red pepper, coarsely chopped
1 c carrots, finely diced or shredded
1 clove garlic, minced
1 c uncooked quinoa
2¼ c sodium-free or low-sodium chicken broth (divided) (I use my homemade chicken broth to as many low-sodium versions contain substantial amounts of sodium.)

Directions
In a skillet, heat 1/4 cup chicken broth until hot. Add vegetables. Cook for 3 to 5 minutes and add quinoa. Cook and stir for 5 more minutes. Add remaining chicken broth. Cover and cook until all the liquid is absorbed, about 20 minutes.

Serves 4

Nutrition Facts
Per Serving: 206 Calories (13% from Fat, 15% from Protein, 72% from Carbohydrate); 8.2 g Protein; 3.0 g Total Fat; 0 g Saturated Fat; 0.1 g Polyunsaturated Fat; 2.4 g Monounsaturated Fat; 37.8 g Carbohydrate; 4.2 g Fiber; 5.4 g Sugar; 365 mg Sodium; 0 mg Cholesterol

Roasted Asparagus

When asparagus is in season, my family loves this dish and asks for it frequently.

Ingredients

20 to 30 spears raw asparagus,5 to 7 inches long
1/2 tbsp extra-virgin olive oil
Pepper to taste

Directions

Preheat oven to 425 degrees. Snap off asparagus bottoms and discard. Place asparagus tops in a bowl and toss with the olive oil and pepper. Lay in a single layer on a baking sheet. Bake for about 10 to 15 minutes.

Serves 4

Nutrition Facts

Per Serving: 38 Calories (39% from Fat, 20% from Protein, 41% from Carbohydrate); 2 g Protein; 1.6 g Total Fat; 0.3 g Saturated Fat;0.1 g Polyunsaturated Fat; 1.2 g Monounsaturated Fat; 4 g Carbohydrate; 2.1 g Fiber; 0 g Sugar; 2.0 mg Sodium; 0 mg Cholesterol

Stir-Fry Vegetables

If you get tired of simply steaming vegetables, try stir-frying them for a welcome change of pace.

Ingredients

1 c raw or frozen broccoli
1 c onion, sliced into strips
1 c carrots, sliced into thin
strips
1 c green pepper, sliced
1 tbsp low-sodium soy sauce,
I use Kikkoman Lite Soy
Sauce
1/2 tbsp cornstarch
1/2 c water

Directions

Mix soy sauce, cornstarch, and water in a small bowl. Heat a skillet or wok over medium-high heat. Add the liquid and cook until hot. Carefully add the vegetables and stir-fry until vegetables are crisp-tender and coated with liquid.

Serves 4

Nutrition Facts

Per Serving: 46 Calories (0% from Fat, 17% from Protein, 83% from Carbohydrate); 2.0 g Protein; 0 g Total Fat; 0 g Saturated Fat; 0 g Polyunsaturated Fat; 0 g Monounsaturated Fat; 10.2 g Carbohydrate; 2.7 g Fiber; 2.6 g Sugar; 173 mg Sodium; 0 mg Cholesterol

Citrus and Honey Sweet Potatoes

Sweet potatoes are a great source of beta-carotene, but if you eat them smothered with marsh-mallows and brown sugar, you add unnecessary calories and sugar. These tasty sweet potatoes will satisfy your sweet tooth without breaking your calorie bank.

Ingredients
2 medium-size sweet potatoes,
    sliced into 1/2-in rounds
1 tbsp brown sugar
3 tbsp organic honey
2 tbsp light margarine such as
    Promise Light
1/2 c orange juice, no pulp
1 tbsp cinnamon

Directions
Preheat oven to 450 degrees. Mix all ingredients together in a rectangular casserole dish. Cover with aluminum foil and bake for about 45 minutes. Test for doneness by sticking a fork into one of the sweet potato rounds. The dish is done if the fork pierces the potato easily.

Serves 4

Nutrition Facts
Per Serving: 163 Calories (14% from Fat, 2% from Protein, 84% from Carbohydrate); 1.4 g Protein; 2.8 g Total Fat; 0.6 g Saturated Fat; 0.4 g Polyunsaturated Fat; 1.3 g Monounsaturated Fat; 35.7 g Carbohydrate; 2.0 g Fiber; 19.5 g Sugar; 53 mg Sodium; 0 mg Cholesterol

Spicy Cucumber Salad

If you love cucumbers, you will appreciate the added kick these seasonings give to them. For an even better flavor, make these one day ahead.

Ingredients
2 c thinly sliced cucumbers
2 tbsp low-sodium Thai fla-
    vored chili sauce
2 tbsp lime juice
1/4 c red onion, finely sliced
4 tbsp fresh cilantro, finely
    diced

Directions
Mix all ingredients together in a medium-size bowl. Serve immediately or refrigerate until dinnertime.

Serves 4

Nutrition Facts
Per Serving: 31 Calories (6% from Fat, 16% from Protein, 78% from Carbohydrate); 1.2 g Protein; 0.2 g Total Fat; 0.1 g Saturated Fat; 0 g Polyunsaturated Fat; 0 g Monounsaturated Fat; 6.1 g Carbohydrate; 1.3 g Fiber; 1.6 g Sugar; 100 mg Sodium; 0 mg Cholesterol

Better Breads and Muffins

Healthy Banana Muffins

I make these muffins in a double or triple batch and freeze them. While I use freshly milled whole wheat, good-quality store-bought whole wheat will give you similar results.

Ingredients

2 c whole-wheat or all-purpose flour
1/4 c granulated sugar (you can combine brown and white sugar if you like)
1 tsp baking soda
1/4 c blackstrap molasses
2 tsp baking powder
1/4 c nuts (optional)
1/2 tsp ground cinnamon
Dash nutmeg
1/4 c ground flaxseed
1 egg or egg substitute
3/4 c skim milk
1/3 c unsweetened applesauce
1/2 tsp vanilla extract
1 c mashed bananas (2 or 3 bananas)

Directions

Preheat oven to 400 degrees. Using a whisk, combine all dry ingredients (flour, sugar, baking soda, baking powder, salt, nuts, and spices) in one bowl. Beat the egg or egg substitute in a small bowl. Whisk the milk, applesauce, and vanilla into the beaten eggs. Pour the wet ingredients into the dry. Fold in the mashed bananas. Divide the batter into muffin pans with paper liners. Cook for 15 to 18 minutes.

Serving: 20 muffins

Nutrition Facts

Per Serving: 90 Calories (10% from Fat, 11% from Protein, 79% from Carbohydrate); 2.5 g Protein; 1 g Total Fat; 0.2 g Saturated Fat; 0.5 g Polyunsaturated Fat; 0.3 g Monounsaturated Fat; 17.7 g Carbohydrate; 2.4 g Fiber; 7.1 g Sugar; 123 mg Sodium; 9.4 mg Cholesterol

Easy Whole-Wheat Yeast Rolls

I make the dough, bake what I need for that evening, and freeze the rest of the dough in 1-inch balls. Thaw the frozen dough balls and bake when they are about doubled in size.

Ingredients

2 packages dry yeast
2 c very warm water
1/4 c Sucanat or 1/3 c honey
1 tbsp salt
1/3 c olive oil
4–5 c whole-wheat flour

Directions

Mix the first five ingredients in the order given. Add 3 1/2 cups flour. Mix well and add the rest of the flour 1/2 cup at a time. Knead by hand for about 10 minutes, adding in extra flour as needed. Put into a bowl and let rise until doubled, or about 60 minutes.

Punch the risen dough down and pull off golf-ball-size pieces of dough. Shape into small balls and place onto a greased baking pan. Cover and allow to rise for about 30 minutes. Bake at 375 degrees until lightly brown, approximately 30 to 40 minutes. Freeze extra rolls for up to three months.

Serving: 24 rolls

Nutrition Facts

Per Serving: 117 Calories (23% from Fat, 10% from Protein, 67% from Carbohydrate); 3.1 g Protein; 3 g Total Fat; 0.5 g Saturated Fat; 0.4 g Polyunsaturated Fat; 2.2 g Monounsaturated Fat; 20 g Carbohydrate; 2.8 g Fiber; 4 g Sugar; 292 mg Sodium; 0 mg Cholesterol

Seven-Grain Bread

This bread is so filling you will probably find it hard to eat too much. A slice counts as one serving.

Ingredients

1 1/3 c warm water (110 degrees F)
2 tbsp vegetable oil
2 tbsp honey
1 tbsp active dry yeast
3 tbsp dry milk powder
2 tsp salt
1 egg
1 c whole-wheat flour
2½ c bread flour
3/4 c seven-grain cereal (I use Kashi 7 Whole Grain Cereal)

Directions

Bread-machine method: Place ingredients in bread machine, starting with the water, olive oil, and honey. Sprinkle flour and cereal on top of the water mixture. Add the remaining ingredients. Remember to keep the yeast, salt, and egg separated before the mixing process begins by making a small well in the center of the flour for the yeast, and placing the salt and egg on opposite sides of the pan. Turn your bread machine on the whole-wheat cycle.

Hand-kneaded method: Place the water, oil, egg, and honey in a bowl. Mix dry ingredients together in a separate bowl. Add about half the flour mixture to the bowl with the wet ingredients and beat with an electric mixer until combined. Add the remaining flour mixture. Beat with the mixer until a sticky dough forms. Turn the dough onto a floured countertop and knead for about 8 to 10 minutes, or until the dough is pliable, stretchy, and soft. Add more whole-wheat flour if needed. Place dough in a lightly greased loaf pan. Cook in a 375-degree oven for about 35 minutes.

Serving: 16 slices

Nutrition Facts

Per Serving: 115 Calories (20% from Fat, 11% from Protein, 69% from Carbohydrate); 3.4 g Protein; 2.5 g Total Fat; 0.3 g Saturated Fat; 0.7 g Polyunsaturated Fat; 1.2 g Monounsaturated Fat; 20 g Carbohydrate; 3.5 g Fiber; 2.5 g Sugar; 300 mg Sodium; 11 mg Cholesterol

Healthy Chicken Choices

Better Than Fried Chicken Fingers

After reading this book, it probably does not surprise you that my children rarely eat fast food. When I make these chicken tenders, I know that all the ingredients are healthy for them. The kids love them, and even though they are a bit high in fat, the fat comes mainly from healthy unsaturated fats.

Ingredients

1 lb thinly sliced chicken breasts or tenders
1/2 c whole-wheat flour
1 c ground almonds
1 tbsp paprika
1/2 tbsp garlic powder (no sodium)
2 tbsp spicy mustard
2 tsp extra-virgin olive oil
1/2 c egg white or egg white substitute

Directions

In a shallow plate or dish, combine the flour, almonds, paprika, garlic powder, mustard, and olive oil. Place the lightly beaten egg whites in a separate shallow bowl. Using gloved hands, coat the chicken breasts in the egg white mixture, then the flour mixture. Place on a baking sheet sprayed with nonstick cooking spray. Bake in a 350-degree oven for 20 to 30 minutes, or until a meat thermometer reads 180 degrees.

Serves: 4

Nutrition Facts

Per Serving: 296 Calories (47% from Fat, 32% from Protein, 21% from Carbohydrate); 24.3 g Protein; 16 g Total Fat; 1.8 g Saturated Fat; 3.6 g Polyunsaturated Fat; 9.7 g Monounsaturated Fat; 15.6 g Carbohydrate; 4.6 g Fiber; 1.2 g Sugar; 69 mg Sodium; 39 mg Cholesterol

Asian-Style Barbecued Chicken

Although I am from the South, I enjoy the spices of Asian dishes. Moving beyond traditional barbecue seasonings, Asian spices take this chicken in a new direction. This dish goes beautifully with brown rice. Adjust your sodium intake for the day you make this dish, as even with low-sodium ingredients, the sodium content is relatively high.

Ingredients

2 tbsp brown sugar
4 tbsp low-sodium soy sauce
2 cloves garlic, finely minced
1 tsp curry powder
2 tbsp low-sodium ketchup
8 chicken thighs or chicken drumsticks, skin removed

Directions

Mix the first five ingredients in a casserole pan to make a marinade. Add the chicken. Spoon the marinade over the chicken until it is completely coated. Marinate for up to 12 hours. Grill outdoors or roast in a 400-degree oven for about 30 minutes.

Serves 6

Nutrition Facts

Per Serving: 344 Calories (35% from Fat, 38% from Protein, 27% from Carbohydrate); 34.7 g Protein; 13.6 g Total Fat; 1.9 g Saturated Fat; 3.1 g Polyunsaturated Fat; 7.3 g Monounsaturated Fat; 23.3 g Carbohydrate; 3.1 g Fiber; 11.4 g Sugar; 669 mg Sodium; 90 mg Cholesterol

Chicken Paprika

*This dish is a family favorite. Spoon the remaining sauce over
whole-wheat egg noodles or brown rice.*

Ingredients
1 tbsp extra-virgin olive oil
1 onion, finely chopped
2–3 cloves garlic, minced
4 boneless, skinless chicken
   breasts
4 tbsp paprika
1 tsp pepper
1 c water

Directions
Heat the olive oil in a large skillet. Add the onion and garlic. Cook until the vegetables are tender and the onions are
almost translucent. Add the chicken to the skillet and sprinkle with paprika and pepper. Allow the chicken to brown
slightly on one side. Then turn the chicken over to brown
the other side. Pour the water into the pan and bring to a
boil. Cover the pan and turn heat down to a simmer. Cook
for 30 to 45 minutes, until the chicken is completely cooked
and tender.

Serves 4

Nutrition Facts
Per Serving: 152 Calories (24% from Fat, 63% from Protein, 13% from Carbohydrate); 24 g Protein; 4.2 g
Total Fat; 0.5 g Saturated Fat; 1 g Polyunsaturated Fat; 2.5 g Monounsaturated Fat; 5 g Carbohydrate; 1.4 g
Fiber; 0.2 g Sugar; 91 mg Sodium; 55 mg Cholesterol

Healthy Chicken Noodle Soup

*A bowl of chicken noodle soup makes a great lunch or dinner dish. When you make your own
soup, you can control the amount of sodium.*

Ingredients
6 c water
2 c homemade, sodium-free
   chicken broth
2 cups of cooked, chopped
   chicken with skin
   removed
1 c chopped carrots
1 c chopped celery
1/2 c chopped white or yellow
   onions
16 oz enriched egg noodles

Directions
Place the water, chicken broth, and raw chicken in a large
saucepot. Bring to a boil and cook until the chicken is completely cooked. Remove the chicken from the pot and set
aside. Add the vegetables to the boiling water and cook for
about 20 minutes or until they are soft. While the vegetables
are cooking, dice the cooked chicken into bite-size pieces.
Add the noodles to the broth and vegetables and cook until
the noodles are tender. Carefully add the diced chicken to the
soup and cook for about 5 minutes. Serve with a side salad
and whole-grain crackers.

Serves 6

Nutrition Facts
Per Serving: 241 Calories (21% from Fat, 51% from Protein, 28% from Carbohydrate); 31 g Protein; 5.5 g
Total Fat; 1.2 g Saturated Fat; 1.2 g Polyunsaturated Fat; 3.0 g Monounsaturated Fat; 16.5 g Carbohydrate;
3.5 g Fiber; 1.6 g Sugar; 30 mg Sodium; 85 mg Cholesterol

Feta and Walnut Chicken Salad

This main-dish chicken salad goes well with whole-wheat rolls and fruit.

Ingredients
2 c cooked chicken breasts, chopped into cubes
8 c shredded romaine lettuce
1 Granny Smith apple, diced
1/4 c black, seedless raisins
1/4 c walnuts
1/4 c crumbled feta cheese
1 c finely sliced red onion
1/4 c balsamic vinegar
1 tbsp extra-virgin olive oil

Directions
In a large bowl, mix all ingredients together. Serve promptly.

Serves 4

Nutrition Facts
Per Serving: 289 Calories (40% from Fat, 33% from Protein, 27% from Carbohydrate); 24 g Protein; 13 g Total Fat; 3.2 g Saturated Fat; 4.7 g Polyunsaturated Fat; 4.7 g Monounsaturated Fat; 20 g Carbohydrate; 4.2 g Fiber; 9.8 g Sugar; 151 mg Sodium; 61 mg Cholesterol

Balsamic-Coated Chicken Breasts

The tang of balsamic vinegar adds interest to an ordinary baked chicken breast.

Ingredients
1 tbsp extra-virgin olive oil
1 lb chicken breasts, bone-in, skinless
1 large red or white onion, sliced
2 cloves fresh garlic, minced
4 tbsp balsamic vinegar
1 c low-sodium chicken broth

Directions
Preheat oven to 375 degrees. Heat the olive oil in a skillet. Add the chicken breasts and brown slightly, turning once. Place the chicken in a casserole dish. In the skillet, cook the onions until they start to brown and get soft. Add the garlic, balsamic vinegar, and chicken broth. Cook for about 5 minutes over medium heat. Once the mixture thickens, pour over the chicken breasts in the casserole dish. Cook in the oven for about 20 to 30 minutes or until the chicken registers 180 degrees on a meat thermometer.

Serves 4

Nutrition Facts
Per Serving: 138 Calories (29% from Fat, 53% from Protein, 18% from Carbohydrate); 18 g Protein; 4.3 g Total Fat; 0.7 g Saturated Fat; 0.5 g Polyunsaturated Fat; 2.7 g Monounsaturated Fat; 5.9 g Carbohydrate; 0.7 g Fiber; 2.0 g Sugar; 205 mg Sodium; 41 mg Cholesterol

Chicken Quesadillas

We love Mexican-inspired food, and these quesadillas appeal to all ages. Using small amounts of reduced-fat cheddar cheese gives you the texture and flavor without the unhealthy saturated fats.

Ingredients

1 c cooked chicken breasts, cut into bite-size cubes
1/2 c cooked black beans
1/2 c salsa
4 tbsp chopped cilantro
4 whole-wheat tortillas, 7 to 8 inches (I use a high-fiber option that has 90 calories and 8 grams of fiber)
Fat-free sour cream as garnish (optional)
Sprinkle of cheddar cheese atop each quesadilla before baking (optional)

Directions

Preheat oven to 375 degrees. Mix all ingredients except the tortillas and sour cream in a mixing bowl. Lay the tortillas on a counter. Place one-quarter of the chicken mixture on one side of each tortilla. Fold the tortillas over the filling. Bake on a flat baking sheet for about 10 to 15 minutes. Serve with fat-free sour cream if desired.

Serves 4

Nutrition Facts

Per Serving: 181 Calories (22% from Fat, 31% from Protein, 47% from Carbohydrate); 14 g Protein; 4.3 g Total Fat; 1.0 g Saturated Fat; 0.4 g Polyunsaturated Fat; 0.6 g Monounsaturated Fat; 21.2 g Carbohydrate; 10.8 g Fiber; 0.6 g Sugar; 374 mg Sodium; 26 mg Cholesterol

Chicken Broccoli Bake

If you have cooked chicken on hand, this dish can be on your table in less than 45 minutes. The chicken broccoli bake reheats well.

Ingredients

1 bunch fresh broccoli
2 c cooked chicken breast, shredded or cubed
1 c coarsely chopped onion
1/2 c reduced-fat cheddar cheese, grated
1 c low-sodium, reduced-fat chicken broth (make your own to reduce the sodium in the dish)
1 cup water
1/4 c plain bread crumbs

Directions

Preheat oven to 350 degrees. Cook broccoli on stove or in microwave until tender. Combine the cooked chicken, onion, cheese, and chicken broth in a large mixing bowl. Add cooked broccoli. Stir well and place into a baking dish. Sprinkle with bread crumbs. Cook for about 20 minutes or until mixture is thoroughly heated.

Serves 6

Nutrition Facts

Per Serving: 267 Calories (21% from Fat, 42% from Protein, 37% from Carbohydrate); 28 g Protein; 6.1 g Total Fat; 1.7 g Saturated Fat; 2.0 g Polyunsaturated Fat; 2.3 g Monounsaturated Fat; 25.2 g Carbohydrate; 10.9 g Fiber; 0.7 g Sugar; 424 mg Sodium; 54 mg Cholesterol

Bruschetta Chicken

This delicious, nutritious dish gives you protein, lycopene, and heart-healthy fats. Although it takes a bit longer to prepare, the extra time is worth the effort.

Ingredients

1 lb chicken breasts, pounded
  to 1/4-in thickness
2 egg whites, lightly beaten
1/2 c Italian bread crumbs
1 c diced fresh tomatoes
1/4 c fresh basil, chopped, or 3
  tbsp dry basil
2 cloves garlic, crushed
1/2 tbsp olive oil

Directions

Preheat oven to 375 degrees. Place the beaten egg whites in a shallow bowl. Combine the bread crumbs, garlic, and basil. Place the dry mixture on a shallow plate. Dredge the chicken breasts in the egg white mixture. Shake off the excess egg white and dredge the chicken in the dry mixture. Place in a 13-by-9-inch casserole dish. Bake for 25 minutes. While the chicken is baking, combine the tomatoes, basil, garlic, and olive oil. After 25 minutes, spoon the tomato mixture onto the chicken. Return chicken to the oven and bake about 10 to 15 minutes more. Chicken is done when a meat thermometer registers 180 degrees.

Serves 4

Nutrition Facts

Per Serving: 246 Calories (18% from Fat, 40% from Protein, 42% from Carbohydrate); 24 g Protein; 5 g Total Fat; 1.5 g Saturated Fat; 1.4 g Polyunsaturated Fat; 1.6 g Monounsaturated Fat; 25.62 g Carbohydrate; 8.9 g Fiber; 1.0 g Sugar; 317 mg Sodium; 40.9 mg Cholesterol

Mexican Chicken Salad

This healthy dish gives you the crunch of the salad greens, the protein in the chicken and beans, and the healthy fats in the avocado. Serve with tortilla chips.

Ingredients

1 lb boneless, skinless chicken
  breasts
1 can sodium-free corn kernels
1 c low-sodium canned black beans
1 diced avocado
2 tbsp lime juice
1/4 c chopped cilantro
1 c tomato, fresh or canned
1/4 c salsa
4 c salad greens, such as romaine or
  a spring mix

Directions

Preheat oven to 400 degrees. Bake chicken in a casserole dish for 20 minutes or until thoroughly cooked. While the chicken cooks, mix corn, black beans, diced avocado, lime juice, cilantro, and tomatoes in a mixing bowl. Cut cooked chicken into thin strips and mix with salsa. Lay salad greens on each individual plate and top with the corn mixture and chicken strips.

Serves 4

Nutrition Facts

Per Serving: 278 Calories (28% from Fat, 37% from Protein, 35% from Carbohydrate); 26 g Protein; 8.7g Total Fat; 1.4 g Saturated Fat; 1.5 g Polyunsaturated Fat; 4.7 g Monounsaturated Fat; 25 g Carbohydrate; 9.4 g Fiber; 1.4 g Sugar; 143 mg Sodium; 49.3 mg Cholesterol

Fabulous Fish

Baked Fish Florentine

This recipe works well with a tender whitefish such as flounder or tilapia.

Ingredients
- 1 lb fish fillets such as flounder
- 8 c raw baby spinach
- 1/4 c fat-free cottage cheese
- 1/4 c Parmesan cheese, freshly grated
- 1 tbsp minced garlic
- 1 c low-sodium tomato juice

Directions

Preheat oven to 375 degrees. Boil the spinach until limp, for 1 to 3 minutes. Dry spinach by rolling the leaves in clean paper towel. Chop spinach into small pieces. Combine cheeses, garlic, and spinach in a small bowl. Lay each fillet on a baking sheet. Place about 1/4 cup of filling in the center of each piece of fish. Roll up each piece of fish. Turn the fish seam side down and secure with a toothpick. Pour the tomato juice over the fish and bake for about 20 minutes.

Serves 4

Nutrition Facts
Per Serving: 214 Calories (18% from Fat, 65% from Protein, 17% from Carbohydrate); 35 g Protein; 4.1 g Total Fat; 1.8 g Saturated Fat; 1.0 g Polyunsaturated Fat; 0.9 g Monounsaturated Fat; 9.2 g Carbohydrate; 1.8 g Fiber; 2.6 g Sugar; 318 mg Sodium; 92.5 mg Cholesterol

Pan-Cooked Salmon with Balsamic Glaze

Salmon gives you healthy fats and loads of protein.

Ingredients
- 12 oz salmon filets, divided into four pieces
- 1 tsp olive oil
- 1 tbsp no-sodium seasoning
- 1/3 c balsamic vinegar
- 1 c orange juice
- 1 tbsp sweet chili sauce
- 4 tbsp chopped basil

Directions

Heat the olive oil and seasoning in a skillet over medium heat. Cook the salmon in the oil and seasoning for about 4 to 6 minutes on each side. Remove the salmon from the pan. Add the vinegar, orange juice, and chili sauce to the skillet. Cook on high heat until the glaze begins to thicken. Add the basil to the glaze, stir to incorporate, and add the salmon back to the pan. Spoon the glaze over the salmon and cook for 1 to 2 minutes.

Serves 4

Nutrition Facts
Per Serving: 450 Calories (27% from Fat, 54% from Protein, 19% from Carbohydrate); 60 g Protein; 13.7 g Total Fat; 3.2 g Saturated Fat; 4.0 g Polyunsaturated Fat; 4.9 g Monounsaturated Fat; 21.7 g Carbohydrate; 2.3 g Fiber; 16.3 g Sugar; 227 mg Sodium; 159 mg Cholesterol

Blackened Cod Tacos

These California-inspired tacos will leave you satisfied and feeling like you just visited a four-star restaurant. You can use red snapper or grouper in place of the cod if you wish.

Ingredients

12 oz cod
1 tbsp sodium-free Cajun spice (omit if your family does not like spicy foods)
1 tbsp canola oil
4 tbsp fat-free sour cream
1 tbsp lime juice
8 flour tortillas (8-in size)
1 tsp cilantro
1 c finely sliced raw cabbage
1/2 c mild or medium salsa

Directions

Heat the canola oil in a skillet until hot. Sprinkle the fish with the Cajun spice, or pepper if you are omitting the spice. Cook the fish for 5 minutes on each side or until completely cooked through. Mix the cilantro with the sour cream and lime juice. Place in the refrigerator. Warm the tortillas in a 350-degree oven for 10 minutes or in the microwave for 30 seconds. Place a small amound of sliced cabbage in each tortilla. Top with the fish fillet. Wrap the tortilla tightly, and spoon the sour cream sauce over each taco.

Serves 4

Nutrition Facts

Per Serving: 239 Calories (27% from Fat, 43% from Protein, 30% from Carbohydrate); 25.5 g Protein; 7.2 g Total Fat; 1.1 g Saturated Fat; 1.3 g Polyunsaturated Fat; 2.2 g Monounsaturated Fat; 17.8 g Carbohydrate; 9.4 g Fiber; 1.8 g Sugar; 422 mg Sodium; 48 mg Cholesterol

Broiled Tilapia with Parmesan Topping

Tilapia is a mild-flavored fish that even non-fish lovers often enjoy. This dish is rather special, but don't let that stop you from serving it to your family as a part of your weekly menu.

Ingredients

12 oz tilapia fillets
4 slices 100 percent whole-wheat bread, reduced calorie
1/4 c finely shredded Parmesan cheese
1 tbsp minced garlic
1 tbsp olive oil
1/4 c chopped fresh parsley
1 tps pepper

Directions

Preheat oven to 400 degrees. Using a food processor, combine the bread slices, cheese, garlic, parsley, and olive oil. Process until finely crumbled. Put the fish on a baking sheet and sprinkle with pepper. Using your hands, pat some of the crumb mixture onto each fish fillet. Bake for about 20 minutes or until fish is flaky and cooked through.

Serves 4

Nutrition Facts

Per Serving: 333 Calories (25% from Fat, 46% from Protein, 29% from Carbohydrate); 38 g Protein; 9 g Total Fat; 1.6 g Saturated Fat; 2.2 g Polyunsaturated Fat; 4.2 g Monounsaturated Fat; 24 g Carbohydrate; 12 g Fiber; 2.2 g Sugar; 312 mg Sodium; 68 mg Cholesterol

Almond-Crusted Fish Sticks

You and your family will enjoy these healthy fish sticks. Serve them with brown or wild rice, a green salad, and berries.

Ingredients
12 oz tilapia, cod, or snapper
1 c plain bread crumbs
1/2 c grated almonds
4 tbsp fat-free mayonnaise
1/4 c skim milk

Directions
Preheat oven to 425 degrees. Mix the bread crumbs and almonds in a shallow dish. Mix the mayonnaise and milk in a separate shallow bowl. Cut the fish into long strips. Dip each strip in the wet mixture, then roll each strip in the bread crumb mixture. Bake the fish sticks for 10 to 15 minutes, until the fish is completely cooked.

Serves 4

Nutrition Facts
Per Serving: 316 Calories (34% from Fat, 35% from Protein, 31% from Carbohydrate); 28 g Protein; 12.3 g Total Fat; 1.4 g Saturated Fat; 3.2 g Polyunsaturated Fat; 6.3 g Monounsaturated Fat; 25 g Carbohydrate; 3.6 g Fiber; 4.4 g Sugar; 274 mg Sodium; 41 mg Cholesterol (Nutritional information based on snapper)

Crab Cakes with Mango Sauce

Don't be intimated by making crab cakes. They are remarkably easy to make and even easier to eat.

Ingredients
1 c crab meat
1 c plain bread crumbs (divided)
4 egg whites or egg white substitute
1 tbsp no-salt seasoning
1/4 c finely diced onion (divided)
1/2 c fat-free Greek yogurt
1 tbsp spicy mustard
1 tbsp low-sodium Worcestershire
   sauce
1 tbsp canola oil
1 c mango, diced into cubes

Directions
Mix the crab, egg whites, 1/2 cup of the bread crumbs, 2 tablespoons of the onion, yogurt, mustard, no-salt seasoning, and Worcestershire sauce in a small bowl. Use your hands to form crab cakes. Combine the remaining bread crumbs and onions. Roll your formed crab cake into the bread crumb and onion mixture. Set on a plate. Heat the canola oil in a small skillet. Cook crab cakes over medium heat. Turn crab cakes once to brown on each side. Top cooked crab cakes with mangos.

Serves 4

Nutrition Facts
Per Serving: 229 Calories (23% from Fat, 29% from Protein, 48% from Carbohydrate); 16 g Protein; 5.6 g Total Fat; 0.7 g Saturated Fat; 1.8 g Polyunsaturated Fat; 2.5 g Monounsaturated Fat; 28 g Carbohydrate; 2.1 g Fiber; 8.8 g Sugar; 226 mg Sodium; 29 mg Cholesterol (Nutritional information based on snapper)

Crispy Fish Sandwich

This fish sandwich will please children and adults. If you do not like flounder,
use tilapia or your favorite whitefish.

Ingredients
12 oz flounder or other whitefish fillets
1 sleeve whole-wheat crackers
1 tbsp spicy mustard
2/3 c whole-wheat flour
4 large egg whites or egg white substitutes
1 tbsp canola oil
4 high-fiber whole-wheat rolls
Lettuce
Sliced tomatoes
Plain Greek yogurt

Directions
Crush the crackers in a food processor or with a rolling pin. Spread each fish fillet with spicy mustard and dredge in whole-wheat flour. Dip the fillets into the egg whites or substitutes, then into the crushed cracker crumbs. Heat the canola oil in a skillet and cook fish for 4 to 6 minutes on each side. Put each piece of cooked fish on a whole-wheat roll spread with Greek yogurt. Top with lettuce and tomatoes.

Serves 4

Nutrition Facts

Per Serving: 289 Calories (7% from Fat, 43% from Protein, 50% from Carbohydrate); 31 g Protein; 2.3 g Total Fat; 0.5 g Saturated Fat; 1.2 g Polyunsaturated Fat; 0.4 g Monounsaturated Fat; 37 g Carbohydrate; 6.1 g Fiber; 1.4 g Sugar; 217 mg Sodium; 57 mg Cholesterol

Garlic Shrimp with Whole-Wheat Pasta

Who doesn't like shrimp? You can prepare this dish quickly, and it will likely disappear off your
dinner plates just as quickly.

Ingredients
1 tbsp olive oil
10 oz raw shrimp
3 cloves garlic, diced
1/4 c fresh parsley
1/3 c lemon juice
Dash salt and pepper
1 c whole-wheat linguine,
    cooked and drained

Directions
Heat oil in a skillet over medium-high heat. Add shrimp and garlic. Cook just until the shrimp turns pink to signal that it is done. Add chopped parsley, lemon juice, salt, and pepper to the skillet. Cook briefly. Serve over cooked pasta.

Serves 4

Nutrition Facts

Per Serving: 268 Calories (16% from Fat, 45% from Protein, 39% from Carbohydrate); 30 g Protein; 4.9 g Total Fat; 0.8 g Saturated Fat; 1.3 g Polyunsaturated Fat; 2.0 g Monounsaturated Fat; 26 g Carbohydrate; 4.1 g Fiber; 1.3 g Sugar; 223 mg Sodium; 110 mg Cholesterol

Baked Salmon

Salmon is easy to bake, and you will be sure to make this sweet-and-sour dish again and again.

Ingredients
12 oz salmon fillets
2 tbsp brown sugar
1 tbsp no-sodium seasoning
1 clove garlic, minced
1/4 c lemon juice

Directions
Preheat oven to 450 degrees. Mix sugar, no-sodium seasoning, and garlic together in a small bowl. Place salmon onto a baking sheet sprayed with nonstick cooking spray. Using gloved hands or a spoon, pat the seasoning mixture onto the fillets. Drizzle lemon juice over the fillets. Bake for 10 to 15 minutes.

Serves 4

Nutrition Facts
Per Serving: 224 Calories (29% from Fat, 39% from Protein, 32% from Carbohydrate); 22 g Protein; 7.1 g Total Fat; 1.1 g Saturated Fat; 2.3 g Polyunsaturated Fat; 2.7 g Monounsaturated Fat; 16 g Carbohydrate; 3.1 g Fiber; 3.1 g Sugar; 167 mg Sodium; 112 mg Cholesterol

Vegetarian Main Dishes

Crispy Black Bean Burritos

A family favorite, this dish is on the menu almost every week. I use dried black beans that I cook myself, but you can substitute low-sodium canned beans.

Ingredients

2 c black beans, cooked at home or
    canned
1/2 tbsp cumin
1/2 tbsp no-sodium seasoning
1/2 tbsp minced garlic
8 tbsp water
1 c chopped tomato
1/4 c sliced green onion
1/2 c shredded, reduced-fat cheddar cheese
4 tortillas (I use high-fiber, whole-wheat ones)

Directions

Preheat oven to 400 degrees. Heat the beans, seasoning, garlic, and water in a sauce pan for 5 minutes. Mash the bean mixture with a potato masher. Spread on tortillas with chopped tomato, green onion, and cheddar cheese. Roll up tortillas and put in a baking dish sprayed with nonstick spray or lined with aluminum foil. Bake for 10 to 15 minutes, until crispy.

Serves 4

Nutrition Facts

Per Serving: 240 Calories (16% from Fat, 30% from Protein, 54% from Carbohydrate); 18 g Protein; 4.3 g Total Fat; 1.4 g Saturated Fat; 0.3 g Polyunsaturated Fat; 0.4 g Monounsaturated Fat; 33 g Carbohydrate; 16 g Fiber; 0.6 g Sugar; 345 mg Sodium; 3 mg Cholesterol

Vegetable and Brown Rice Paella

Getting my kids to eat a variety of vegetables is easier when I use a lot of different vegetables. With quick-cooking brown rice, you can have this meal ready in just a few minutes.

Ingredients

1 c asparagus
1/2 tbsp minced garlic
1 c chopped green bell pepper
1 c sliced onion
4 c spinach
1 chopped tomato
1 c chopped zucchini
1 tbsp no-sodium seasoning
1 c cooked brown rice
1/4 c sliced almonds, toasted in the oven

Directions

Place 1/4 cup of water into a skillet. Heat the skillet until the water is hot. Toss in the vegetables and seasoning. Cook until the vegetables are crisp-tender. Add cooked rice to the vegetables and cook for 3 minutes. Divide among four plates and top with a sprinkle of toasted almonds.

Serves 4

Nutrition Facts

Per Serving: 144 Calories (25% from Fat, 17% from Protein, 68% from Carbohydrate); 6.6 g Protein; 4 g Total Fat; 0.4 g Saturated Fat; 1.1 g Polyunsaturated Fat; 2.1 g Monounsaturated Fat; 24 g Carbohydrate; 5.2 g Fiber; 2.3 g Sugar; 34 mg Sodium; 0 mg Cholesterol

Vegetarian Frittata

This frittata loses the calories associated with most frittatas but retains the flavor and protein from the egg substitutes. This dish is perfect for a summer evening meal.

Ingredients
1 tbsp olive oil
1 c asparagus spears
1 c sliced red onion
1 c sliced zucchini
1 c halved cherry or grape tomatoes
1 tbsp no-sodium seasoning
2 c egg substitute (from the freezer or dairy section)
1 oz finely shredded Parmesan cheese

Directions
Preheat oven broiler. In an ovenproof skillet on the stove, cook asparagus, onion, zucchini, and tomatoes in olive oil for about 5 minutes. Sprinkle with seasoning mix. Pour egg substitute into the skillet and mix until it begins to set. Add Parmesan cheese to the top, place skillet under the broiler, and cook for 5 minutes or until the frittata is completely set.

Serves 4

Nutrition Facts
Per Serving: 295 Calories (28% from Fat, 28% from Protein, 44% from Carbohydrate); 21 g Protein; 9.4g Total Fat; 2.1 g Saturated Fat; 1.5 g Polyunsaturated Fat; 5.2 g Monounsaturated Fat; 33 g Carbohydrate; 7.5 g Fiber; 3.9 g Sugar; 304 mg Sodium; 6.1 mg Cholesterol

Baked Spinach Linguine

If you use whole-wheat pasta, this is a terrific, low-fat way to get healthy grains into your diet.

Ingredients
10 oz whole-wheat linguine
1/2 c reduced-fat mozzarella cheese
10 oz chopped, frozen spinach
4 tbsp fat-free sour cream
1/4 c egg substitute or 1 whole egg
1 tbsp Italian seasoning
2 cloves garlic, minced
16 oz low-sodium spaghetti sauce
2 tbsp reduced-fat Parmesan cheese

Directions
Preheat oven to 350 degrees. In a large stockpot, bring about 3 quarts water to a boil. Add whole-wheat pasta, stirring to prevent sticking. While pasta is cooking, mix the cheese, thawed and drained spinach, sour cream, egg or egg substitute, seasonings, and garlic in a 9-by-13-inch casserole pan. Drain the cooked pasta and pour it into the casserole pan. Mix thoroughly. Top with spaghetti sauce and sprinkle with Parmesan cheese. Bake for 45 to 60 minutes or until completely heated through.

Serves 8

Nutrition Facts
Per Serving: 253 Calories (27% from Fat, 27% from Protein, 46% from Carbohydrate); 17 g Protein; 7g Total Fat; 2.4 g Saturated Fat; 1.3 g Polyunsaturated Fat; 3.3 g Monounsaturated Fat; 29.4 g Carbohydrate; 5.9 g Fiber; 2.6 g Sugar; 243 mg Sodium; 8.6 mg Cholesterol

Blender Gazpacho

This refreshing gazpacho fills you up with a variety of vegetables and loads of flavor. I like to serve it with grilled chicken breasts, and a loaf of whole wheat bread.

Ingredients

4 medium tomatoes, quartered
1 medium seedless cucumber, peeled and roughly chopped (about 2 to 2½ c)
1 small red bell pepper, chopped (about 3/4 to 1 c)
1 tbsp sherry vinegar
2 cloves garlic, peeled

Directions

Place all ingredients in a blender or food processor. Blend until completely smooth. Divide the soup among six small bowls and serve with your favorite whole-wheat bread.

Serves 6

Nutrition Facts

Per Serving: 30 Calories (12% from Fat, >1% from Protein, 88% from Carbohydrate); 1.2 g Protein; 0.4 g Total Fat; 0.1 g Saturated Fat; 0.1 g Polyunsaturated Fat; 0 g Monounsaturated Fat; 6.6 g Carbohydrate; 1.5 g Fiber; 1.4 g Sugar; 8.9 mg Sodium; 0 mg Cholesterol

My Famous Black Beans and Rice

Well, this dish may not be famous worldwide, but my secret ingredient gives it a kick that most black bean dishes seem to miss.

Ingredients

16 oz dried black beans or 3 cans sodium-free black beans, drained
1/2 c water
3 c chopped fresh tomatoes
1/2 c chopped green pepper
1/2 c chopped onions
1/4 c white vinegar
1/4 c cooked brown rice per person

Directions

Prepare the black beans according to the package directions or drain canned beans. Place beans, water, tomatoes, green pepper, and onions in a large saucepan. Bring to a boil and simmer over low heat for about 30 minutes. Add vinegar after 30 minutes and cook for 5 more minutes. Serve over brown rice.

Serves 6

Nutrition Facts

Per Serving: 152 Calories (7% from Fat, 20% from Protein, 73% from Carbohydrate); 7.8 g Protein; 1.2 g Total Fat; 0.2 g Saturated Fat; 0.5 g Polyunsaturated Fat; 0.2 g Monounsaturated Fat; 28 g Carbohydrate; 8.1 g Fiber; 2.4 g Sugar; 19 mg Sodium; 0 mg Cholesterol

Oven "Fried" Eggplant

This is a twist on a recipe I found in Cooking Light magazine. Although my family doesn't gener-ally love eggplant, everyone gave this dish a thumbs-up.

Ingredients

6 oz fat-free Greek yogurt, plain flavor
1 tbsp finely minced red onion
1 lb unpeeled eggplant, sliced into 1/2-in slices
1/3 c low-sodium bread crumbs
1/4 c low-fat Parmesan cheese
1 tbsp Italian seasoning

Directions

Combine Greek yogurt and red onion in a small bowl. Dip each eggplant slice into the yogurt and onion mixture, coating well on both sides. In a small shallow dish, combine the bread crumbs, Parmesan cheese, and Italian seasoning. Dip the coated eggplant in the crumb mixture. Place the eggplant in a single layer on a large baking sheet. Cook for about 12 to 15 minutes, turn the eggplant over once, and cook another 15 minutes. Serve over whole-wheat pasta and marinara sauce.

Serves 6

Nutrition Facts

Per Serving: 349 Calories (17% from Fat, 23% from Protein, 60% from Carbohydrate); 15 g Protein; 4.4 g Total Fat; 1.7 g Saturated Fat; 1.0 g Polyunsaturated Fat; 0.9 g Monounsaturated Fat; 52 g Carbohydrate; 16 g Fiber; 5.6 g Sugar; 189 mg Sodium; 4.9 mg Cholesterol

Tomato and Onion Quiche

You can make this crustless quiche ahead of time and cook it later in the day. I serve it with a salad topped with grilled chicken, whole-wheat rolls, and fruit.

Ingredients

2–3 tomatoes, cut into 1/4-in-thick slices
1/2 c chopped white or yellow onion
3 eggs or 3/4 c egg substitute
3/4 c skim milk
1/8 cup all-purpose flour
1 tbsp fresh basil or 1 tsp dried basil
1/4 tsp dry mustard
1/4 tsp pepper
1/4 c reduced-fat Swiss or Colby-Jack cheese

Directions

Preheat oven to 425 degrees. Place tomato slices onto clean paper towel for a few minutes to absorb the extra moisture. While the tomatoes rest, heat 1 to 2 table-spoons of water in a small skillet. Add the onion to the skillet, cooking until translucent. Remove from heat when done. In a small mixing bowl, whisk together eggs, skim milk, flour, and seasonings. Spoon onions into the egg mixture. Slowly pour onion and egg mixture into a pie plate sprayed with nonstick cooking spray. Lay sliced tomatoes on top of the egg mixture. Sprinkle with cheese and bake for about 45 minutes.

Serves 6 to 8

Nutrition Facts

Per Serving: 90 Calories (17% from Fat, 23% from Protein, 60% from Carbohydrate); 9 g Protein;1.5 g Total Fat; 0.9 g Saturated Fat; 0.1 g Polyunsaturated Fat; 0.1 g Monounsaturated Fat; 9.9 g Carbohydrate; 1.5 g Fiber; 2.6 g Sugar; 129 mg Sodium; 5.1 mg Cholesterol (Nutrition information based on using egg substitutes.)

Better Beef Dishes

Grilled Flank Steak

We do not eat beef, but in my beef-eating days, I frequently used flank steak because of its lean properties and ease of cooking.

Ingredients

Marinade:
1/4 c low-sodium teriyaki sauce
1 tbsp red wine vinegar
2 tsp low-sodium Worcestershire sauce
2 tsp minced garlic
1/8 tsp hot red pepper sauce
1 (15 oz) boneless, lean flank steak

Sherry sauce:
1 tbsp reduced-calorie margarine
1/4 c finely chopped red onion
2 oz dry sherry
2 tsp Dijon mustard
2 tsp cornstarch
1 c low-sodium or sodium-free beef broth

Directions

Combine all marinade ingredients and marinate flank steak for 8 to 12 hours. Spray broiler pan or grill with nonstick cooking spray. Remove flank steak from marinade and broil or grill steak for 15 to 20 minutes, or until done to your preference.

Prepare sauce by melting the reduced-calorie margarine in a skillet and sautéing the onion until soft. Stir in the sherry and mustard and cook for about 5 minutes. In another bowl, mix cornstarch with a few tablespoons of beef broth. Stir, and add in the remaining broth. Pour mixture into the saucepan and cook until it begins to thicken.

Pour over the cooked steak and serve with a green salad.

Serves 4

Nutrition Facts

Per Serving: 277 Cal (34% from Fat, 52% from Protein, 14% from Carbohydrate); 33 g Protein; 10 g Total Fat; 4 g Saturated Fat; 1.8 g Polyunsaturated Fat; 4 g Monounsaturated Fat; 9 g Carbohydrate; 0 g Fiber; 4 g Sugar; 28 mg Calcium; 3 mg Iron; 365 mg Sodium; 58 mg Cholesterol

Spaghetti Sauce with Lean Ground Beef

When I make spaghetti sauce, I use vegetarian crumbles. But lean ground beef works equally well and gives meat lovers a healthy, satisfying, and low-fat sauce.

Ingredients

8 oz lean ground beef
1/2 c chopped onion
3 cloves garlic, finely minced
28 oz crushed tomatoes (no-salt variety)
12 oz no-salt tomato paste
2–3 tbsp Italian seasoning

Directions

Brown lean ground beef, onions, and garlic in a skillet. Cook completely. Drain fat from ground beef mixture and pat with clean paper towel to remove more fat. Add tomatoes, tomato paste, and Italian seasoning to the mixture. Bring to a boil and simmer on low for about 30 minutes. Stir frequently to prevent burning.

Serves 6 to 8

Nutrition Facts

Per Serving: 183 Calories (32% from Fat, 28% from Protein, 40% from Carbohydrate); 14 g Protein; 7 g Total Fat; 3 g Saturated Fat; 0.8 g Polyunsaturated Fat; 3 g Monounsaturated Fat; 20 g Carbohydrate; 5 g Fiber; 11 g Sugar; 68 mg Calcium; 4 mg Iron; 70 mg Sodium; 31 mg Cholesterol

Filet Mignon with Vegetable Kabobs

Filet mignon is pricey, but it is a lean cut of beef. Keep your servings small to keep your calories low.

Ingredients

1 lemon, zested and juiced
1 tbsp extra-virgin olive oil
1 tbsp dried oregano
1/4 tsp freshly ground pepper
12 cherry tomatoes
10 oz white mushrooms, stemmed
1 medium zucchini, halved
    lengthwise and sliced into
    1-in pieces
1 small red onion, cut into wedges
1 12-oz piece of filet mignon
    steak, 1½–2 in thick, cut into
    4 pieces

Directions

Preheat outdoor grill to high. Combine lemon zest and juice, olive oil, oregano, and pepper in a large bowl. Reserve 2 tablespoons of marinade in a small bowl. Add tomatoes, mushrooms, zucchini, and onion to the remaining marinade; toss well to coat. Thread vegetables onto eight 10-inch wooden skewers that have been soaked in water for about 20 minutes. Drizzle skewers and filet mignon with the reserved marinade.

Grill steak 4 to 6 minutes per side for medium and 6 to 8 minutes per side for medium-well done. Grill vegetable kababs for about 8 to 12 minutes. Turn skewers frequently to avoid burning vegetables.

Serves 4

Nutrition Facts

Per Serving: 221 Calories (35% from Fat, 48% from Protein, 17% from Carbohydrate); 27 g Protein; 9 g Total Fat; 3 g Saturated Fat; 2.2 g Polyunsaturated Fat; 3 g Monounsaturated Fat; 10 g Carbohydrate; 3 g Fiber; 3 g Sugar; 33 mg Calcium; 4 mg Iron; 58 mg Sodium; 71 mg Cholesterol

Southwest Sloppy Joes

These are sure to please you and your family. Use the leanest ground beef you can find, and put only 3 ounces in each pita half to ensure your calories stay low.

Ingredients

1 lb extra-lean ground beef or 1 lb
    ground turkey
1/2 c chopped green pepper
1 garlic clove, minced
1 tbsp chopped onion
3/4 c low-sodium barbecue sauce
1/2 c no-salt corn kernels, drained
1/4 c chopped green chilies
1/2 tsp no-sodium seasoning
4 whole-wheat pita pockets, split in half

Directions

Place ground beef, green pepper, garlic, and onion into a medium-size skillet. Cook over medium heat until beef is completely cooked through. Drain any fat. Add barbecue sauce, corn, chilies, and seasoning. Bring to a boil. Reduce heat to low and simmer for about 15 minutes. Spoon 3 ounces of Sloppy Joe mixture into each pita half.

Serves 8

Nutrition Facts

Per Serving: 241 Calories (14% from Fat, 34% from Protein, 52% from Carbohydrate); 21 g Protein; 4 g Total Fat; 1 g Saturated Fat; 1.3 g Polyunsaturated Fat; 1.2 g Monounsaturated Fat; 32 g Carbohydrate; 3 g Fiber; 9 g Sugar; 254 mg Sodium; 43 mg Cholesterol

Delectable Desserts

Peach Granola Crisp

You can make this dish with fresh peaches, frozen peaches, or peaches canned in their own juice. Avoid syrup-sweetened peaches.

Ingredients

1 c low-fat or fat-free granola (Try Kellogs's Low-Fat Granola)
1/4 c brown sugar or Sucanat, loosely packed
1/2 tsp cinnamon
1 tbsp reduced-calorie margarine, melted
4 c peaches
1/2 c water
1 c fresh strawberries or raspberries (optional)

Directions

Preheat oven to 350 degrees. In a small mixing bowl, combine granola, brown sugar, and cinnamon. Drizzle with melted reduced-calorie margarine. Mix with a fork until mixture appears crumbly. Mix peaches with water and place in a square casserole dish. Top with granola mixture. Bake for about 10 minutes or until granola is slightly browned. Top with berries, if desired.

Serves 6

Nutrition Facts

Per Serving: 166 Calories (16% from Fat, 6 from Protein, 88% from Carbohydrate); 2.5 g Protein; 3.1 g Total Fat; 0.9 g Saturated Fat; 0.7 g Polyunsaturated Fat; 1.3 g Monounsaturated Fat; 36.5 g Carbohydrate; 4.2 g Fiber; 14 g Sugar; 68 mg Sodium; 2.1 mg Cholesterol

Easiest Sorbet Ever

This dessert is so simple that I hesitated to put it in the book. But my family loves it, and I think yours will too.

Ingredients

1 cup of canned fruit packed in its own juice (generally about 2 cans). (We use peaches, pears, or pineapples.)

Directions

Remove fruit from the cans and place in a freezer-safe bowl. Freeze overnight. Remove from freezer, place in blender, and process until smooth. Serve immediately.

Serves 4

Nutrition Facts

Per Serving: 165 Calories (13% from Fat, 5% from Protein, 82% from Carbohydrate); 2.4 g Protein; 2.4 g Total Fat; 0.7 g Saturated Fat; 0.6 g Polyunsaturated Fat; 1.0 g Monounsaturated Fat; 34 g Carbohydrate; 4.5 g Fiber; 11 g Sugar; 58 mg Sodium; 1.5 mg Cholesterol

Chocolate-Banana Milkshake

I am a big fan of chocolate. This dessert should definitely be reserved for the occasional treat. A fun variation on this recipe is to replace the vanilla extract with 1/2 teaspoon of peppermint extract.

Ingredients
1 c skim milk
3 tbsp dark chocolate syrup
1/2 c fat-free chocolate yogurt
    or ice cream
2 bananas, frozen
2 tsp vanilla extract

Directions
Combine all five ingredients in a blender and process until smooth. Serve in small cups or bowls.

Serves 2

Nutrition Facts
Per Serving: 227 Calories (3% from Fat, 13% from Protein, 84% from Carbohydrate); 7.3 g Protein; 0.8 g Total Fat; 0.4 g Saturated Fat; 0.1 g Polyunsaturated Fat; 0.2 g Monounsaturated Fat; 47.8 g Carbohydrate; 2.4 g Fiber; 34 g Sugar; 98 mg Sodium; 5.0 mg Cholesterol

Chocolate Chip Meringues

These are light and fluffy and can satisfy your craving for a sweet, low-calorie dessert. They are relatively high in sugar, so eat just one at a time.

Ingredients
3 egg whites
1 c sugar
1 tbsp vanilla
6 tbsp unsweetened cocoa
    powder
3 tbsp dark chocolate chips

Directions
Preheat oven to 200 degrees. Spray a foil-lined baking sheet with non-stick spray. Mix egg whites with an electric mixer until soft peaks begin to form. Slowly add in sugar and vanilla. Beat further until stiff peaks begin to form again. With a plastic spatula, fold in cocoa powder and mini choco-late chips. Use a spoon to drop 1 teaspoon at a time onto the baking sheet. Bake for 45 minutes, until the cookies are lightly browned and crispy. Cool completely before eating. Store in a tightly covered container.

Serves 12 (2 cookies per serving)

Nutrition Facts
Per Serving: 133 Calories (11% from Fat, 8% from Protein, 81% from Carbohydrate); 2.7 g Protein; 1.6 g Total Fat; 1.0 g Saturated Fat; 0 g Polyunsaturated Fat; 0.2 g Monounsaturated Fat; 28 g Carbohydrate; 1.5 g Fiber; 24 g Sugar; 32 mg Sodium; 0.8 mg Cholesterol

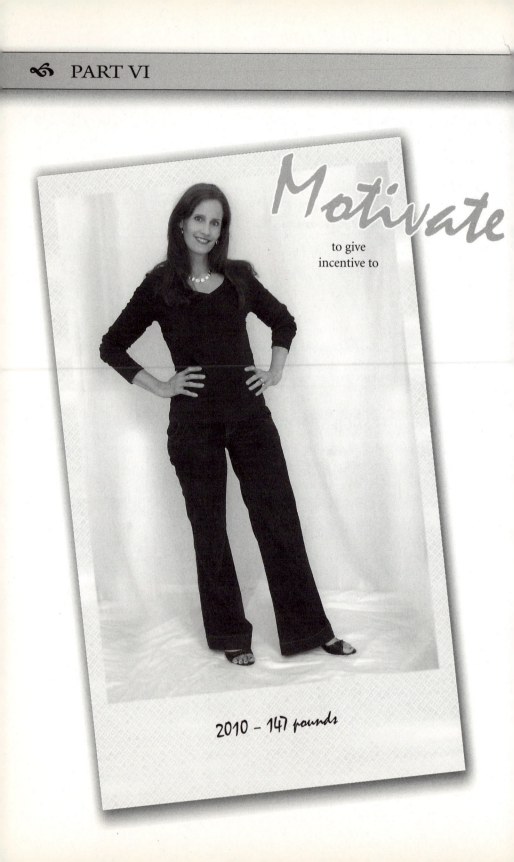

PART VI

Motivate

to give
incentive to

2010 - 147 pounds

Exercises

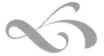

Exercise is a key component to achieving a healthy lifestyle, as exercise offers you both health and weight-loss benefits. In the following section, I outline two twelve-week walking programs. One is for beginning walkers. The other is for those at an intermediate level.

In addition, I include a wide variety of strength-training exercises for you to choose from. The exercises cover your upper body, lower body, and core muscles. Use the exercise log in appendix K to record your workouts. Over time, you will likely enjoy analyzing how much your fitness level has improved.

Note: Before beginning any exercise routine, get evaluated by a physician.

Twelve-Week Walking Program for Beginning Exercisers

Begin with the exercise routine for week 1, shown below. If fifteen minutes is not enough of a workout for you, move to week 2. Continue moving forward until you reach a level where you get winded during your workout but are not totally exhausted. Stand up straight when you walk, look straight ahead, and keep your lower arms parallel to the ground. Gently tighten your abdominal muscles to avoid slouching.

Walk three times each week for the first four weeks, then increase to four or five times each week. Repeat weeks as you feel the need. Once you reach week 12, work on increasing your speed to cover more distance and burn more calories in the same time period.

Make copies of the exercise worksheet in appendix K to keep track of your walking workouts and to monitor your progress.

Week	Warm-up (minutes)	Intense Walking (minutes)	Cool Down (minutes)	Total Walking Time (minutes)
1	3	5	5	13
2	5	6	5	16
3	5	9	5	19
4	5	12	5	22
5	5	15	5	25
6	5	18	5	28
7	5	20	5	30
8	5	22	5	32
9	5	25	5	35
10	5	28	5	38
11	5	31	5	41
12	5	34	5	44

Twelve-Week Intermediate Walking/Speed Walking Workout

Begin this walking program if you have completed the beginner workout or already consistently walk for exercise. Focus on walking as briskly as possible during the intense walking phase. The faster you walk, the more calories you will burn. Focus on form by holding yourself straight, walking from heel to toe, and taking short, fast steps.

Repeat weeks as many times as needed. You may find that once you reach week 5, you need to do each week twice to build up your endurance.

Week	Warm-up (minutes)	Intense Walking (minutes)	Cool Down (minutes)	Total Walking Time (minutes)	Frequency
1	5	15	5	25	3 times per week
2	5	18	5	28	3 times per week
3	5	20	5	30	4 times per week
4	5	23	5	33	4 times per week
5	5	26	5	36	5 times per week
6	5	29	5	39	4 times per week
7	5	32	5	42	5 times per week
8	5	36	5	46	4 times per week
9	5	39	5	49	5 times per week
10	5	42	5	52	4 times per week
11	5	46	5	56	4–5 times per week
12	5	50	5	60	4–5 times per week

Strength-Training Exercises You Can Do at Home

Most of the exercises described below involve dumbbells or your body weight. Some require an exercise ball. When using dumbbells, use 2-pound weights in the beginning and add more weight each month. Aim for ultimately lifting 5 to 10 pounds or a weight that challenges you.

Upper-Body Exercises

Dumbbell Rows

Stand by an armless chair or low bench. Place your lower left leg and left hand on the chair or low bench. Hold a dumbbell in your right hand, keeping your arm almost straight. Hold your back in a straight line, inhale, and pull the dumbbell straight up toward the ceiling. Exhale and slowly lower the dumbbell back to its original position. Repeat eight times. Rest briefly and do eight more lifts. Switch sides and perform the exercise with your left arm.

Muscles worked: upper back, shoulders

Triceps Kickbacks

Start in the same position as the dumbbell row, with the dumbbell in your right hand. Instead of letting the arm hang straight down, bend it at a 90-degree angle. Inhale and move the hand with the weight straight toward the wall behind you. Stop when your elbow is almost straight. Hold for 1 second and return your arm to its original position. Perform two sets of eight repetitions on each side.

Muscles worked: triceps

Easier Push-ups

Kneel on a carpeted floor or exercise mat. Place your hands in front of you, so they are positioned slightly wider than your shoulders. Adjust your knees until your upper body is suspended in the air and your back is straight. Tighten your abdomen, inhale, and lower your upper body. Stop when your chest is about 2 to 3 inches from the floor. Exhale and push your body back to the starting position. Begin with five push-ups. Add two to three push-ups every week until you can do twenty-five push-ups in this position.

Muscles worked: arms, shoulders, chest, abdomen

Advanced Push-ups

A standard military-style push-up, the advanced push-up requires you to support yourself with just your toes and hands while lowering and raising your body. Keeping your abdominal muscles tight will help keep your body and back from sagging.

Muscles worked: arms, shoulders, chest, abdomen

Bicep Curls

This classic exercise begins with you standing straight and tall. Hold a dumbbell in each hand, with your wrists facing away from your thighs. Your feet should be about shoulder distance apart. Inhale and lift one dumbbell toward your shoulder. Hold briefly and lower your hand. Repeat with the other hand. Repeat eight times with each hand. Then repeat the sequence one or two more times. Keep your abdominal muscles tight to avoid arching your back as you lift the weights. Concentrate on keeping your elbows tucked right into your side as you lift and lower the dumbbells.

Muscles worked: biceps

Dumbbell Flies

You can do this exercise on a low wooden bench or exercise bench. Lie on your back on the bench. Hold a dumbbell in each hand. Bend your elbows to bring your arms to a 90-degree angle. Your wrists should be facing your head. Lift your arms in the air, keeping your wrists straight. Stop when your elbows are almost locked. Hold and lower your arms back to their starting position. Repeat two or three sets of eight repetitions.

Muscles worked: pectorals, shoulders

Preacher Curls with an Exercise Ball

Prepare for the curl by placing two medium-weight dumbbells on the floor. Put your exercise ball close to the dumbbells. Kneel behind the ball and lie over it with your upper body. Keep your upper thighs in contact with the ball. Grab the dumbbells with your inner wrists facing away from you. Lift the dumbbells toward the ceiling. Make sure that your upper arms stay on the ball. Repeat eight to twelve times, rest, and then perform the sequence again.

Muscles worked: biceps

Wrist Curls with a Dumbbell

Sit on a sturdy chair with one heel touching the chair leg and the other heel about 1 foot away from the chair leg. Hold a dumbbell in the hand on the side of the slightly extended leg. Resting your elbow on your leg, slowly lower your hand until your wrist and upper arm is parallel to the floor. Exhale and curl your wrist toward your body. Inhale and lower your wrist. Repeat eight times with each wrist.

Muscles worked: forearms

Hammer Curls

Hammer curls are another biceps exercise. Stand with your legs about shoulder distance apart, holding a dumbbell in each hand. Keep your shoulders back and your arms extended. Your wrists should be facing your outer thighs. Lift the dumbbells straight up, stopping when the dumbbells are close to your shoulders. Slowly lower the dumbbells. Repeat eight times. Repeat one more set of eight lifts.

Muscles worked: biceps

Upright Dumbbell Rows

Stand with your feet slightly more than shoulder distance apart. Engage your core muscles by tightening your abdominal muscles and standing up straight to keep from arching your back. Hold a dumbbell in each hand. Begin with your arms straight down. Make sure your inner wrists are facing the front of your thighs. Exhale and lift the up toward the ceiling, keeping the dumbbells close to your body. Stop when the dumbbells are about even with your collarbones. Inhale and lower the weights. Do two repetitions of eight lifts.

Muscles worked: shoulders, upper back

Lower-Body Exercises

Wall Squats with an Exercise Ball

Stand near a solid wall. Place an exercise ball between your lower back and the wall. Position the ball so that it is snuggled securely next to your lower back. Keep the ball from falling down by leaning against the wall. Maneuver your feet so they are about 1 foot from the wall. Inhale and bend your knees and hips as you lower your buttocks toward the floor. You should feel like you are about to sit in a chair. At first, do not lower yourself more than a few inches. As you get stronger, lower your body until your upper thighs are almost parallel to the ceiling and your knees are bent at a 90-degree angle. Repeat eight to twelve times.

Caution: Do not allow your knees to go beyond your toes as you lower your body.

Muscles worked: quadriceps, hamstrings, glutes

Modified Lunges

This is a good lunge exercise for beginners. Stand near a wall in case you need to grab something for support. Stand with your feet slightly apart. Pull your body up tall by tightening your abdominal muscles. Take a step slightly longer than your normal walking step. Shift your weight to the leg you just walked forward on. Lower your body slowly, bending your hips and both knees at the same time. Keep your weight on your heels rather your toes. Keeping your heels on the ground will help you keep your front knee from bending past your front toe. Whenever you perform lunges, your knee should be slightly behind your toe to help protect your knee from injury. Hold for a second and push back up, returning to your upright position. Repeat eight to ten times on each leg. Work up to two sets per session.

Muscles worked: glutes, quadriceps

Walking Lunges

Perform walking lunges after you are very comfortable with modified lunges. This exercise requires a long open space such as a hallway or large room. Stand with your feet slightly apart. Hold your arms by your sides or place your hands on your waist for balance. Inhale as you take a long step forward with your right leg. Lower your body as you place your right foot, so that your knees are bent and your right thigh is parallel to the ceiling. Push your body back to your starting position using your legs and step forward with your left leg. Repeat for eight to twelve steps.

Muscles worked: quadriceps, glutes, abdominal muscles, hamstrings

Single Leg Raise (Lying)

Lie on your back on the floor. Extend your legs straight and point your toes at the ceiling. Bend your right knee and slide your right foot back toward your buttocks. Stop when your knee is slightly bent and your foot is flat on the floor. Push your lower back into the floor. Raise your left leg straight into the air. Try to get your leg up to about a 45-degree angle. At first you may be able to lift your leg only a few inches. Hold for two to three seconds and gently lower your leg. Repeat eight times on each leg, then do one more round.

Muscles worked: quadriceps

Calf Raises

This easy exercise strengthens and defines your calf muscles. Stand on an exercise step or the lowest step of your stairs at home. Step up with your right foot. As your foot touches the step, rise up on your toes like a ballet dancer. Hold yourself in this upright position for two to three seconds. Lower your heel and step back off the step. Do eight to ten sets on each foot.

Muscles worked: calves

Leg Extensions while Seated

You can do this exercise at the office or at home. Sit on a supportive chair, with your feet flat on the floor and your back away from the chair's back. Place your hands on either side of your thighs and hold the edge of the chair. Exhale and lift your right foot off the floor a couple of inches. Extend your right knee until your leg is close to parallel to the floor. Hold for one to two seconds and then lower your leg. Do five to eight lifts with each leg.

Muscles worked: quadriceps

Hamstring Curls with an Exercise Ball

Place an exercise ball on a carpeted floor or mat. Lie face down on the floor, with your legs near your exercise ball. Maneuver the ball so it is between your calves. Squeeze the ball tightly with your lower legs. Your hands should be under your chin. Exhale and lift the ball by curling your heels toward your lower body. Keep lifting as far as possible, keeping your upper thighs in contact with the floor. Lower the ball and repeat eight times. Rest and do one more repetition.

Muscles worked: inner thighs and hamstrings

Forward Lunges with a Dumbbell

Do this exercise after you are comfortable with lunges without a dumbbell. Stand with your legs about 12 inches apart. Hold a dumbbell in each hand, with your inner wrist facing your outer thigh. Inhale while taking a long step forward with your left leg. Keep your upper body very straight by tightening your abdominal muscles. As you take the step, allow both of your knees to bend. Lunge down until your upper thigh is close to parallel with the ceiling and your right knee is close to the floor. Exhale as you push up with your left leg and return to your starting position. Repeat eight times on your left leg, rest briefly, and then do the lunges with your right leg leading.

Muscles worked: quadriceps, glutes

Bridges on Ball

Sit on your exercise ball. Once you are stable, walk your feet forward, allowing the ball to roll under your body. Stop when your feet are about 3 feet from the ball and your upper/mid-back is the only part of your upper body touching the ball. Your buttocks should be about 6 to 8 inches from the floor. Exhale, push your hips toward the ceiling, and allow the ball to roll back slightly until your mid- to lower back is supported by the ball. Hold the position, keeping your upper thighs parallel to the ceiling. Inhale and return to your starting position. Repeat eight times.

Muscles worked: hamstrings, glutes

Core and Abdominal Exercises

Crunches

You can't go wrong with the basic crunch for a good overall strengthening exercise. Lie on your back on a firm floor. Bend your knees. Keep your feet slightly apart and flat on the floor. Place your hands near each ear, with your elbows extending away from your head. Exhale and lift your shoulders and upper back off the floor. Inhale and roll your upper back and head back to the floor. Repeat ten times. Rest and repeat twenty more times, as you are able.

Muscles worked: abdomen

Crunches on an Exercise Ball

Doing crunches on a ball helps stabilize your back while giving you a great core workout. Sit on your ball. Roll the ball under your buttocks and lower back by walking your feet away from the ball. Keep walking until your lower back is right on the upper curve of the ball. Place your hands by your ears and lift your shoulders toward the ceiling by tightening your abdominal muscles. Roll your shoulders back down. Repeat twenty times.

Muscles worked: abdomen

Planks

Start this challenging exercise with your knees on the ground, as with the modified push-up, or by supporting yourself with just your toes, forearms, and hands. Kneel on your hands and knees. Push your legs behind you until your body is long and straight. Balance your upper body on your hands and forearms and lift your entire body off the floor. Your back should be straight, with your neck and head in alignment with your spine. Hold the position for ten seconds. Release and try again. Do not let your back sag.

Muscles worked: abdomen, core muscles

Superman

Lie face down on an exercise mat. Extend your arms straight above your head, as though you are going to dive into a pool. Extend your legs straight and keep your feet, knees, and ankles together. Engage your abdominal muscles and lift your upper and lower body off the floor at the same time. Hold for a few seconds, rest, and repeat two to five more times.

Muscles worked: abdomen, lower back

Standing Side Bend

Stand with your legs slightly more than hip-width apart. Hold a rolled-up towel or exercise band between your hands. Lift your arms above your head as though you are going to perform a jumping jack. Visualize lifting your upper body toward the ceiling and lean about 12 inches to your right. Hold for two seconds, return to the starting position, and then bend to your left. Repeat twelve times.

Muscles worked: oblique abdominal muscles

Appendix A

Practice Problems for Calculating Fat Percentage

Fat percentage formula:

Calories from fat divided by calories per serving equals total percentage of fat

Problem 1
Food item: hummus
Serving size: 2 tbsp
Calories per serving: 54
Calories from fat: 24

What is the fat percentage of hummus? _____

Problem 2
Food item: frosted shredded wheat
Serving size: 24 biscuits
Calories per serving: 203
Calories from fat: 8

What is the fat percentage of frosted shredded wheat? _____

Problem 3
Food item: pancakes from a mix
Serving size: 2 pancakes
Calories per serving: 300
Calories from fat: 34

What is the fat percentage of pancakes from a mix? _____

Problem 4
Food item: hamburger bun
Serving size: 1 bun
Calories per serving: 114
Calories from fat: 18

What is the fat percentage of a hamburger bun? _____

Problem 5
    Food item: frozen chicken pot pie
    Serving size: 1/2 frozen pie
    Calories per serving: 314
    Calories from fat: 168

    What is the fat percentage of frozen chicken pot pie? _____

Problem 6
    Fat-free Greek yogurt
    Serving size: 6 oz
    Calories per serving: 140
    Calories from fat: 0

    What is the fat percentage of fat-free Greek yogurt? _____

Problem 7
    Food item: couscous prepared with seasonings and 1/2 tbsp olive oil
    Serving size: 1/2 c
    Calories per serving: 120
    Calories from fat: 66

    What is the fat percentage of couscous with seasonings and olive oil? _____

Problem 8
    Food Item: Alfredo sauce made with skim milk
    Serving size: 1/2 c
    Calories per serving: 79
    Calories from fat: 18

    What is the fat percentage of Alfredo sauce made with skim milk? _____

Problem 9
    Food Item: chicken and broccoli with bowtie pasta
    Serving size: 3/4 c
    Calories per serving: 196
    Calories from fat: 40

    What is the fat percentage of chicken and broccoli with bowtie pasta? _____

Problem 10
    Food Item: fast-food French fries
    Serving size: small
    Calories per serving: 230
    Calories from fat: 99

    What is the fat percentage of fast-food French fries? _____

Answers

1.

$24 \div 54 = .44$

Hummus has 44 percent of its calories from fat. Hummus is a healthy, low-calorie snack with healthy fats. Just watch the portion size.

2.

$8 \div 203 = .039$

Frosted shredded wheat has just 3.9 percent of its calories from fat. Shredded wheat is a healthy cereal, with a low fat and a high fiber content.

3.

$34 \div 300 = .11$

Pancakes have 11 percent of their total calories from fat. Pancakes are a good choice, provided you do not take away the nutritional value by adding large quantities of syrup. Instead of syrup, top pancakes with fresh chopped fruit.

4.

$18 \div 114 = .158$

Hamburger buns have about 15.8 percent of their calories from fat. Hamburger buns are fine to eat. For better health, choose ones made from whole grains or whole wheat.

5.

$168 \div 314 = .535$

Chicken pot pie has about 53.5 percent of its calories from fat. Chicken pot pie looks healthy, but between the cream, butter, and pie crust, it is not the best choice.

6.

$0 \div 140 = 0$

This one is too easy for an explanation. Zero fat and loads of calcium and protein make Greek yogurt a great choice.

7.

$66 \div 120 = .55$

Couscous prepared with olive oil has about 55 percent of its calories from fat. Couscous by itself is low fat, but when prepared with too much oil, it can become a high-fat food.

8.

$18 \div 79 = .23$

Alfredo sauce prepared in a healthy way has about 23 percent of its calories from fat. If prepared properly, Alfredo sauce can be a nice change from standard tomato-based sauces.

9.

$40 \div 196 = .20$

Chicken and broccoli with pasta has about 20 percent of its total calories from fat. This is a tasty combination and a healthy choice, especially if you use whole-wheat pasta.

10.

$99 \div 230 = .43$

A small serving of French fries has 43 percent of its calories from fat. While tasty, French fries are not the best choice when you are trying to lose weight. They are high in fat and sodium and lack nutrients.

Appendix B

Fat Percentages

Calories and Fat Percentages in Common Foods

As you look at this list, you may be surprised that almost all foods have some fat, even spinach and romaine lettuce. Do not avoid foods with fat; just learn to choose foods with healthy fats, such as vegetables, fruits, grains, lean meats, healthy oils, and fat-free dairy.

Food	Serving Size	Calories	Fat Percentage
Apple cinnamon oatmeal	1 packet	128	11
Oat bran bagel	1 3½-in bagel	268	4
Scrambled eggs	2 eggs	182	66
Diet whole-wheat bread	2 slices	91	10
Oat bran muffin	1 medium	305	25
Multigrain cereal	1 c	110	8
Fast-food hamburger	1 small	279	44
Provolone cheese	1 slice	98	68
Tomato	1 tomato	22	10
Veggie burger	1 patty	97	24
Potato chips	1 oz	160	56
Grapes	1 c	62	5
Apple	1 medium	95	3
Pretzels	1 oz	108	8
Brownie	2-in square	112	56
Sweet potato	1 medium	103	less than 1
Avocado	1 c	234	82 (healthy fats)
Roasted chicken breast	1 c	231	19
Broccoli	1 c	31	10
Brown rice	1 c	216	7
Dry-heat-cooked salmon	1/2 fillet	367	54
Lean ground beef	3 oz	196	47
Quinoa	1/2 c	111	14
Egg McMuffin	1 muffin	300	36
Orange	1 medium	85	2
Olive or canola oil	1 tbsp	120	100
Romaine lettuce	1 c	8	16
Raw spinach	1 c	7	15
Almonds	23 almonds	162	72

Source: USDA Nutrient Data Laboratory

Appendix C

Pocket Guide for Fat Calorie Limits

To learn whether a food has less than 30 percent of its calories from fat, multiply calories per serving by .30. Compare the result to the listing for calories from fat. Below, I have done some of the math for you. Keep a copy of this list in your purse or wallet to use when shopping. If calories from fat are higher than the number listed, proceed with caution!

Calories Per Serving		Recommended Maximum Fat Calories
90	x 30%	27
100	x 30%	30
110	x 30%	33
120	x 30%	36
130	x 30%	39
140	x 30%	42
150	x 30%	45
160	x 30%	48
170	x 30%	51
180	x 30%	54
190	x 30%	57
200	x 30%	60
210	x 30%	63
220	x 30%	66
230	x 30%	69
240	x 30%	72
250	x 30%	75
260	x 30%	78
270	x 30%	81
280	x 30%	84
290	x 30%	87
300	x 30%	90

Note: While it is good to limit your daily food choices to foods that have 30 percent or less of their calories from fat, some healthy foods exceed the 30 percent limit. Examples are nuts, olive oil, flaxseeds, and fish. These foods should be a part of your diet (see chapter 3).

Appendix D

BMI Chart

Weight	Height								
	58	59	60	61	62	63	64	65	66
	4' 10"	4' 11"	5' 0"	5' 1"	5' 2"	5' 3"	5' 4"	5' 5"	5' 6"
100	21	20	20	19	18	18	17	17	16
105	22	21	21	20	19	19	18	18	17
110	23	22	22	21	20	20	19	18	18
115	24	23	23	22	21	20	20	19	19
120	25	24	23	23	22	21	21	20	19
125	26	25	24	24	23	22	22	21	20
130	27	26	25	25	24	23	22	22	21
135	28	27	26	26	25	24	23	23	22
140	29	28	27	27	26	25	24	23	23
145	30	29	28	27	27	26	25	24	23
150	31	30	29	28	27	27	26	25	24
155	32	31	30	29	28	28	27	26	25
160	34	32	31	30	29	28	28	27	26
165	35	33	32	31	30	29	28	28	27
170	36	34	33	32	31	30	29	28	27
175	37	35	34	33	32	31	30	29	28
180	38	36	35	34	33	32	31	30	29
185	39	37	36	35	34	33	32	31	30
190	40	38	37	36	35	34	33	32	31
195	41	39	38	37	36	35	34	33	32
200	42	40	39	38	37	36	34	33	32
205	43	41	40	39	38	36	35	34	33
210	44	43	41	40	38	37	36	35	34
215	45	44	42	41	39	38	37	36	35
220	46	45	43	42	40	39	38	37	36
225	47	46	44	43	41	40	39	38	36
230	48	47	45	44	42	41	40	38	37
235	49	48	46	44	43	42	40	39	38
240	50	49	47	45	44	43	41	40	39
245	51	50	48	46	45	43	42	41	40
250	52	51	49	47	46	44	43	42	40
255	53	52	50	48	47	45	44	43	41
260	54	53	51	49	48	46	45	43	42
265	56	54	52	50	49	47	46	44	43
270	57	55	53	51	49	48	46	45	44

If you like to figure things out for yourself, the calculation for BMI is: weight in pounds times 703, divided by height in inches. If you're not a math whiz, here is the chart:

67	68	69	70	71	72	73	74	75	76
5' 7"	5' 8"	5' 9"	5' 10"	5' 11"	6' 0"	6' 1"	6' 2"	6' 3"	6' 4"
16	15	15	14	14	14	13	13	13	12
16	16	16	15	15	14	14	14	13	13
17	17	16	16	15	15	15	14	14	13
18	18	17	17	16	16	15	15	14	14
19	18	18	17	17	16	16	15	15	15
20	19	18	18	17	17	17	16	16	15
20	20	19	19	18	18	17	17	16	16
21	21	20	19	19	18	18	17	17	16
22	21	21	20	20	19	19	18	18	17
23	22	21	21	20	20	19	19	18	18
24	23	22	22	21	20	20	19	19	18
24	24	23	22	22	21	20	20	19	19
25	24	24	23	22	22	21	21	20	20
26	25	24	24	23	22	22	21	21	20
27	26	25	24	24	23	22	22	21	21
27	27	26	25	24	24	23	23	22	21
28	27	27	26	25	24	24	23	23	22
29	28	27	27	26	25	24	24	23	23
30	29	28	27	27	26	25	24	24	23
31	30	29	28	27	27	26	25	24	24
31	30	30	29	28	27	26	26	25	24
32	31	30	29	29	28	27	26	26	25
33	32	31	30	29	29	28	27	26	26
34	33	32	31	30	29	28	28	27	26
35	34	33	32	31	30	29	28	28	27
35	34	33	32	31	31	30	29	28	27
36	35	34	33	32	31	30	30	29	28
37	36	35	34	33	32	31	30	29	29
38	37	36	35	34	33	32	31	30	29
38	37	36	35	34	33	32	32	31	30
39	38	37	36	35	34	33	32	31	30
40	39	38	37	36	35	34	33	32	31
41	40	38	37	36	35	34	33	33	32
42	40	39	38	37	36	35	34	33	32
42	41	40	39	38	37	36	35	34	33

Appendix E

Calorie-Counting Worksheet

Date: _____

Time	Servings	Food	Calories	Fat %
			Total	

Water (8 oz per circle)
O O O O O O O O O O O

Appendix F

Weekly Food Diary

Day 1

Breakfast	Lunch	Dinner	Snacks

Day 2

Breakfast	Lunch	Dinner	Snacks

Day 3

Breakfast	Lunch	Dinner	Snacks

Day 4

Breakfast	Lunch	Dinner	Snacks

Day 5

Breakfast	Lunch	Dinner	Snacks

Day 6

Breakfast	Lunch	Dinner	Snacks

Day 7

Breakfast	Lunch	Dinner	Snacks

Appendix G

Weekly Menu Planning Worksheet

Sunday	Date:
Breakfast	
Lunch	
Snacks	
Dinner	
Side	
Side	
Side	
Monday	Date:
Breakfast	
Lunch	
Snacks	
Dinner	
Side	
Side	
Side	
Tuesday	Date:
Breakfast	
Lunch	
Snacks	
Dinner	
Side	
Side	
Side	
Wednesday	Date:
Breakfast	
Lunch	
Snacks	
Dinner	
Side	
Side	
Side	

Thursday	Date:
Breakfast	
Lunch	
Snacks	
Dinner	
Side	
Side	
Side	
Friday	Date:
Breakfast	
Lunch	
Snacks	
Dinner	
Side	
Side	
Side	

Notes

Grocery List

❏	❏
❏	❏
❏	❏
❏	❏
❏	❏
❏	❏
❏	❏
❏	❏
❏	❏
❏	❏
❏	❏
❏	❏

Appendix H

Ten Low-Fat, Low-Calorie Eating Tips

1. Examine meat and trim off all visible fat before broiling, grilling, or baking.

2. When roasting vegetables or meats, coat them with 1 teaspoon extra-virgin olive oil. I pour 1 teaspoon into my gloved hand and rub the food with the oil, rather than pouring it out of the bottle. Olive oil gives you healthy fats.

3. Avoid salting your food. Use fresh herbs from your garden, buy quality dried herbs and seasonings, or purchase fresh herbs from the produce section of your grocery store. Once you give your palette a break from extreme salt, you will be surprised how much fresher food tastes.

4. Ditch the full-fat milk, yogurt, and cream. Wean yourself off full-fat milk by combining it with a little 1 percent or skim milk in your glass or cereal bowl. Over time, add more low-fat milk and less high-fat milk. You will be eating less saturated fats and calories.

5. Pop your own popcorn in an air popper. A 2 1/2-cup serving of air-popped popcorn has about 3 grams of fiber and almost no fat. Avoid buttered microwave popcorn, movie popcorn, and popcorn cooked in a lot of oil.

6. Train yourself to think of fruit in the evening as dessert. Over time, you won't miss cakes or pies, and when you do have a piece, you will appreciate it as a treat.

7. Substitute homemade or low-calorie commercially prepared hummus for high-fat mayonnaise in egg salads, chicken wraps, or any other dish you traditionally make with mayonnaise.

8. Switch your toast topping from butter or margarine to either fresh fruit spread or a butter-flavored spread that contains plant sterols. Plant sterols can help your cholesterol levels.

9. Fill up your dinner plate with vegetables first instead of filling your plate with heaping mounds of pasta or several dinner rolls. Vegetables are super low in calories and full of vitamins and minerals.

10. After you boil chicken, put the broth in the refrigerator overnight. In the morning, skim any fat off the broth. Freeze the broth in 1-cup freezer-safe containers. Chicken broth is a great substitute for oil when sautéing vegetables. Or use it instead of highly salted canned broths.

Appendix I

Healthy Meal and Snack Ideas

It's nice to have a list of meal and snack ideas that you can turn to when nothing sounds good. Add your own ideas on the blank lines at the end of each section.

Breakfast Ideas
- Breakfast burritos using whole-wheat wraps
- Egg white omelets
- Oatmeal with fresh fruit
- Steel-cut oats (when you have time to let them cook) (recipe on page 234)
- Banana bran muffins made with whole-wheat flour (recipe on page 240)
- Whole-grain cereal with skim milk
- Fruit parfait layered with Greek yogurt, fresh fruit, and a sprinkle of nuts
- Whole-wheat toast topped with 100 percent fruit spread

Add your own ideas here:

_____

_____

_____

_____

_____

_____

_____

_____

_____

_____

Lunch Ideas

- Homemade broth-based soups such as minestrone and vegetable
- Spinach, chicken, and hummus wraps
- Tuna salad made with canned light tuna, Greek yogurt, and organic celery
- Chicken sandwiches made from leftover chicken. Add a homemade low-sodium barbecue sauce
- Green salad with a variety of vegetables, 1 ounce of feta cheese, five olives, and lemon juice
- Veggie burgers on whole-wheat, low-calorie buns
- Grilled turkey breast sandwiches with mustard, sauerkraut, and apple slices

Add your own ideas here:

_____

_____

_____

_____

_____

_____

_____

_____

_____

_____

_____

_____

Dinner Ideas

- Green salad topped with cubed, grilled chicken and cooked white beans, seasoned with balsamic vinegar
- Quick homemade pizzas made with low-sodium tomato sauce and fresh herbs. Top with vegetables and sprinkle with part-skim mozzarella cheese.
- Your choice of meat grilled indoors or outdoors. Serve with baked sweet potato, grilled vegetables, and fruit.

- Vegetarian chili made with red kidney beans, vegetarian meat substitute, and your favorite chili vegetables
- Grilled salmon or tilapia served with a fresh salad and topped with lemon juice
- Breakfast for dinner: scrambled eggs or egg substitute with sautéed tomatoes and green peppers; serve with whole-wheat toast, a fruit salad, and a side of Greek yogurt
- Black beans and rice
- Vegetarian lasagna

Add your own ideas here:

_____

_____

_____

_____

Snack Ideas
- 1 ounce unsalted roasted almonds
- Frozen banana on a stick
- Fruit kebob
- Fresh veggies with Greek yogurt or hummus dip
- Boiled egg
- Two cups of air-popped popcorn
- Fruit and yogurt smoothies
- Cottage cheese topped with red and green peppers
- Two graham crackers topped with 2 teaspoons natural, low-calorie peanut butter
- Celery spread with hummus
- Small box of raisins and fifteen lightly salted peanuts
- Low-fat cheese stick and two ounces of nitrate-free turkey

Add your own ideas here:

_____

_____

_____

Appendix J

Grocery List Template

Produce (vegetables, fruits)	
❏	❏
❏	❏
❏	❏
❏	❏

Dry Goods (cereal, rice, pasta, oatmeal)	
❏	❏
❏	❏
❏	❏
❏	❏

Canned Goods (fruit, low-salt soup, vegetables, tuna)	
❏	❏
❏	❏
❏	❏
❏	❏

Breads/Baking Items (bread, buns, flour, mixes, yeast)	
❏	❏
❏	❏
❏	❏
❏	❏

Refrigerated Foods (lean meat, poultry, cheese, milk, low-fat yogurt)	
❏	❏
❏	❏
❏	❏
❏	❏

Frozen Foods (vegetables, meat, desserts, juice, pizza)	
❏	❏
❏	❏
❏	❏
❏	❏

Snacks/Drinks (coffee, tea, juice, crackers, nuts, diet drinks)	
❏	❏
❏	❏
❏	❏
❏	❏

Condiments/Spices (mustard, mayonnaise, syrup, peanut butter, jelly, pepper, dressing)	
❏	❏
❏	❏
❏	❏
❏	❏

Household Goods (paper towels, tissues, plastic bags, cleaning supplies)	
❏	❏
❏	❏
❏	❏
❏	❏

Baby/Pet Supplies (diapers, wipes, pet food)	
❏	❏
❏	❏
❏	❏
❏	❏

Miscellaneous	
❏	❏
❏	❏
❏	❏
❏	❏
❏	❏
❏	❏
❏	❏
❏	❏
❏	❏
❏	❏
❏	❏

Appendix K

Weekly Workout and Exercise Log

Date:	Start Time:	End Time:
Weight:	Hours of Sleep:	

Fitness Goal (strength, muscle building, fat loss, endurance, other):

Body Parts Trained (check all that apply)
❑ Whole Body ❑ Chest ❑ Back ❑ Shoulders ❑ Legs ❑ Calves ❑ Biceps ❑ Triceps ❑ Abs ❑ Other:

Cardio, Aerobic, or Conditioning Exercise

Exercise	Time/Distance/Intensity/Speed/Calories	Notes

Weight, Strength, and Resistance Training

Exercise	Weight	Sets	Reps	Rest	Notes

Diet and Nutrition

Meal	Foods Eaten/Ingredients	Approximate Calories
Preworkout		
Postworkout		

Workout Rating (1 to 10):

Workout Notes to Yourself

Index

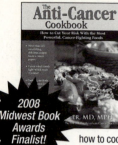
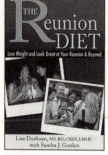
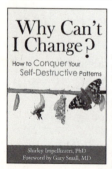